Chair Yoga

Balance With Gentle Chair-based Exercises

(A Guide to Revitalize Mind & Body With Gentle Exercise)

Albert Edwards

Published By **Ryan Princeton**

Albert Edwards

Chair Yoga: Balance With Gentle Chair-based Exercises (A Guide to Revitalize Mind & Body With Gentle Exercise)

ISBN   978-1-998038-18-3

No part of this guidebook shall be reproduced in any form without permission in writing from the publisher except in the case of brief quotations embodied in critical articles or reviews.

Legal & Disclaimer

The information contained in this book is not designed to replace or take the place of any form of medicine or professional medical advice. The information in this book has been provided for educational & entertainment purposes only.

The information contained in this book has been compiled from sources deemed reliable, and it is accurate to the best of the Author's knowledge; however, the Author cannot guarantee its accuracy and validity and cannot be held liable for any errors or omissions. Changes are periodically made to this book. You must consult your doctor or get professional medical advice before using any of the suggested remedies, techniques, or information in this book.

Table Of Contents

Chapter 1: What is yoga and how might it benefit me?

Yoga has long been practiced in India as an ancient and intricate technique to support physical and mental growth. While it began as a simple ritual, its popularity has grown over time as an effective means for managing daily challenges.

Yoga as commonly taught in the US typically consists of authentic positions (asanas), breathing techniques (pranayama), and self-assessment (Dyana).

Yoga styles range from sensitive practices to demanding ones, and research studies often contrast these types of yoga. Therefore, it is difficult to define which benefits yoga has on achievement without further study.

Yoga and two Chinese shows of skill -- kendo and qi gong -- are often described as "shrewd new turn of events" practices. Each of the three practices incorporates both clever parts and genuine ones.

Sherwin emphasizes the significance of association in understanding yoga, which derives from Sanskrit (regarded as the essential language of yoga).

According to her, this is an appropriate way of portraying yoga, given all that's happening today. "We show it as connecting the mind and body through breath," she states.

Sherwin emphasizes the many advantages of yoga, noting it as a form of personal development. But yoga is much more than that: "Yoga is an entire lifestyle; positions are only one part of it," she states. "Yoga has become part of their everyday lives."

Yoga originated in India and has been practiced for nearly 5,000 years, according to Sherwin. "Initially it was taught one-on-one and only to those of great status," she explains.

At its core, yoga serves to foster achievement on all levels - physical, mental, basic, and striking.

Yoga has not yet been subjected to widespread condemnation, according to The Yoga Connection. It can be practiced and respected by people of all beliefs, from realists and pundits alike.

History of Yoga

Yoga's approach to encounters often lacks definition and require reflection on its oral transmission, its inclined toward texts and models' befuddling thoughts. The early works on yoga were unraveled on sensitive palm leaves which were unfortunately damaged or lost over time; some experts even speculate that yoga could be up to 10,000 years old! Today we can trace its development back through four seasons of progress, practice and refinement.

Yoga Before Standard Deviations

The indus-Sarasvati human progress of Northern India laid the foundations of Yoga long before today. The word itself was first mentioned in one of India's oldest sacred texts, The Device Veda. The Vedas were sacred texts containing melodies, mantras and customs used by Brahmans - the Vedic clergymen - for worship. Yoga was perfected and perfected by the Brahmans and Rishis (mystic diviners), who revealed their practices and convictions in the Upanishads, an expansive work with over 200 widely-favored texts. One of the most influential Yogic game plans is the Bhagavad-Gita, written around 500 B.C.E. The Upanishads took this challenge and created something truly remarkable: they showed penitence for one's mental self through self-data, action (karma yoga) and knowledge (jnana yoga).

Old Style Yoga

Prior to the advent of Patanjali's Yoga-Sutras, yoga practiced was an eclectic jumble of different beliefs and methods that often clashed or clashed. His text "Yoga-Sutras," the foundational text for modern RAJA YOGA (commonly referred to as "standard yoga") provided an orderly systematization of poses and stages leading up to Samadhi or illumination - making him widely regarded as the father of modern yoga; its teachings still influence most styles today.

Post-Standard Yoga

A long time after Patanjali, yoga experts developed practices designed to restore the body and bring out life. They disregarded the depictions of ancient Vedas and accepted that our bodies could be an asset in reaching light. Through Tantra Yoga, moderate ways of thinking were employed to cleanse both mind and body of any restrictions or barriers that hinder us from being true to ourselves. This evaluation led directly to what is now commonly known as Hatha Yoga in Western culture today.

The Present-Day Period

Yoga practitioners began making an impact in the late 1800s and mid-1900s, spreading out across America with students as their ally. At the 1893 Parliament of Religions in Chicago, Expert Vivekananda mesmerized attendees with his lectures on yoga and the diversity of world religions. In the 1920s and 30s, Hatha Yoga gained unparalleled prominence in India due to T. Krishnamacharya, Expert Sivananda, and other yogis who practiced it. Krishnamacharya founded the pioneering Hatha Yoga school in Mysore in 1924, and Sivananda established the Incomparable Life Society on the banks of the sacred Ganges River two decades later. Krishnamacharya left behind three students that would continue his legacy and spread Hatha Yoga: B.K.S. Iyengar, T.K.V. Desi achar and Pattabhi Jois. Sivananda was an influential essayist who authored over 200 books on yoga as well as founding nine ashrams around the world to spread its reach.

Yoga began to spread westward gradually until Indra Devi opened her Hollywood yoga studio in 1947. Since then, more western and Indian educators have joined in on the fun, developing hatha yoga further and winning over new followers. Soon enough, there were multiple schools or styles of hatha yoga popping up around the world with various emphasises on different parts of preparation.

Importance and Benefits of Yoga

Over the past decade, there has been an exponential rise in yoga's acceptance. Clinical-trained experts and celebrities alike are endorsing its many advantages. But while some may view yoga as just another broad game plan that incorporates new age divination techniques, others find it quite alienating; what they don't understand is that what they perceive as another course of action won't provide them with the results they had hoped for.

Before exploring the potential benefits of Yoga, it's essential to comprehend its true essence. Yoga is not a religion but an approach for managing everyday existence that encourages mental clarity in a physically healthy body - as taught by Ayurveda in India. While certain actions such as extreme exercises may enhance wellbeing in some way or another, they have no real effect on improving one's basic or astral body.

Yoga isn't just about doing poses or holding your breath. It is an intentional practice designed to bring you into a state of awareness wherein you accept reality as it exists and let go, allowing the material body to become luxurious and contented with itself - this ties in with yoga's goal of uniting all things as one. That is the connection made possible through this union created through yoga: experiencing yourself as part of the universe while feeling one with it all; this is its effect on you.

Yoga was first taught by Patanjali, who famously said: "Sthiram sukham asanam." This means a place that feels firm and free is your asana. Yet an asana is only the first step on your journey towards true self-awareness -

in other words: yoga revolves around celebrating harmony within yourself so everything works in sync for maximum benefit. When you allow yourself to change so everything fits perfectly inside, you will unlock all your capabilities.

Hatha Yoga and its various branches (Ashtanga Yoga, Iyengar Yoga, Bikram Yoga, Yin Yoga, Kundalini Yoga) can all provide harmony for you during preparation depending on what you enjoy and the issues that need addressing.

Normal progressions of yoga practice encompass:

*Further makes frontal cortex limit

*Lower impressions of tension

*Changes quality explanation

*Increasing versatility

*Hacks downbeat

*Further creates lung limit

*Works with fretfulness

*Moves unsurprising back torture

*Further develops the energy of balance
*More grounded bones

*Strong weight

Yoga reduces the risk of heart illnesses

Yoga as a status symbol has immense benefits that affect an individual both physically and psychologically. From decreasing your pulse to increasing torment resistance, there are multiple things yoga does for you that you might not realize:

Further Developed Course:

Yoga helps strengthen your bloodstream, leading to improved oxygen transportation throughout the body. Furthermore, an improved circulation system reveals healthier organs and radiant skin.

Further Develops Position:

Yoga provides guidance on how to maintain control and transform. With regular practice, your body will recognize the correct position, giving off an image of calm assurance.

Hoists Your Personality:

Yoga allows you to hoist yourself up onto a pedestal. Through regular practice you'll develop awareness about yourself as an individual - hoisting up whatever attributes make up your personality!

Consistent yoga practice can enliven your spirit and invigorate you in a moment as it fills your body with revitalizing energy.

Chapter 2: Yoga Fosters Harmony

Yoga not only seeks to foster harmony within you, but it also helps you manage your body. A typical demonstration of yoga will challenge you to switch positions within the class and focus well outside it.

Organ Awareness:

Yoga strengthens your internal organs, providing extra protection from contaminations. After spending so much time cultivating yourself physically and mentally, you'll know immediately if something doesn't feel quite right when practicing yoga.

Extended Safety:

Yoga and resistance have long been associated. As yoga works to recover and develop each cell in your body, your immunity increases significantly - ultimately strengthening it for longer-lasting protection against external threats.

Imbuing Full Body Care:

Exercising yoga for everyday reasons will help you become aware of your own body. With time, yoga helps you make small but significant changes that will transform how you approach life. At the end of it all, yoga helps you feel good about yourself!

Improvement of Gastrointestinal Prosperity:

Regular yoga practice helps to stimulate the stomach-related system and clear away other stomach ailments like indigestion or gas. Gastroscopic abilities are beneficial to people of all ages; learn more about acid reflux home fixes for improved wellness.

Extending Center Strength:

It's essential to recognize when your middle is solid for you, body solid for you. Your middle holds all of your body's weight, helping build assurance from wounds and aiding recovery more quickly. Yoga works in the middle, making it sound, versatile and strong.

More Raised Degrees of Anguish Strength:

Yoga helps build resistance against torture and takes steps toward relieving intense suffering.

Extended Absorption:

Yoga places strict limitations on processing in order to achieve healthy absorption - essential for reaching one's ideal weight.

Further-Developed Sexuality: Yoga encourages all individuals to discover their sexual potentials.

Yoga builds your bravery and offers total surrender while giving you more control. This gives your sexuality a vital lift.

Restored Energy:

Yoga can restore both mind and body to their original states of equilibrium. People who practice yoga on a regular basis report feeling enabled after each gathering of poses.

Additionally, it creates rest:

Yoga helps you decompress your mind, release any unnecessary tensions, and get more rest.

Composed Capacity of the Body:

Yoga implies congruity. When you practice yoga for everyday reasons, your mind starts working in collaboration with your body - leading to further improvement and magnificence.

Licenses Self-Affirmation:

Yoga encourages care and growth toward success. Your assurance grows, making you more certain.

Builds Self-Control:

Yoga shows you the best way to express caution in all areas of life.

Restores an Inspiring Perspective:

Yoga helps restore and strengthen many aspects of our tactile framework, giving us a renewed perspective of reality. Consequently, when yoga is practiced regularly, many more neural connections are made. This makes you more confident and allows us to look at things from an elevated standpoint.

Diminishing Enmity:

When yoga is performed for everyday purposes, the shock is greatly reduced. Through breathing and examination, yoga calms the physical framework, decreasing irritation and hostility. A decline in hostility also indicates a reduction in circulatory strain - leading to a serene approach towards life that encourages better decision-making.

Improve Concentration:

Consistent yoga practice will eventually bring about the best obsession, and after two to two months of consistent practice, you should find yourself more prodded and focused than ever before.

Quietness and Serenity:

As you breathe deeply and think clearly, it helps you relax your perspective. Standard yoga practice enables perfection to become part of who you are - not just a piece of preparation. With regular practice, perfection becomes part of everyday life!

Today yoga has become accessible to people of all ages and backgrounds, with no age limitations. Its presence around the globe has become part of everyday life for some individuals and thanks to modern technology it allows yogis and educators to share their expertise more readily than ever before.

Does Yoga Count as Exercise?

Although yoga wasn't originally created to be an exercise program, certain styles have evolved into practices focused on the true aspects of preparation, according to Edward Laskowski MD - a genuine prescription and reclamation expert and former co-director of Mayo Office Sports Drug in Rochester, Minnesota. "People come into yoga with different goals in mind; some may enjoy the intellectual aspect while others need more significant amounts of action and development."

Dr Laskowski emphasizes the importance of keeping our heartbeat elevated during anticipation for periods of increased wellbeing. "The heart is a muscle," he states, and when you challenge it by raising your pulse rate, it helps keep it more grounded."

Laskowski believes yoga isn't quite on par with running or traveling when it comes to aerobic activities, but the amount of oxygen-consuming benefit an individual could gain depends on the style and pace of their practice, according to Laskowski.

Chapter 3: Clinical Benefits of Yoga

Laskowski emphasizes that "the benefits of yoga vary for each individual," noting its potential to aid with adaptability, strength, socialization and endurance." She adds:

Research has demonstrated that mindfulness can assist with an array of outcomes, including weight loss and support, as well as cardiovascular wellness.

An analysis of one year's late evaluation results found that individuals who practiced yoga experienced improvements across several dimensions of flourishing, such as fear, stress, body structure, heartbeat rate, aggravation level and metabolic markers for those with type 2 diabetes.

A meta-assessment revealed that yoga mediations could assist individuals with BMI of 25 or higher to reduce their pulse. The benefits were greatest when the yoga intercession included breathing strategies and reflection.

According to another survey, yoga motivated 66% of individuals to practice more regularly and 40% to improve their eating habits.

There is evidence to support the idea that yoga may provide benefits to individuals with chronic illnesses and infections, physical torment or other adverse impacts, as well as overall satisfaction.

Vinyasa Yoga

Jen Fleming, a yoga educator and supervisor at Yoga Works in Atlanta, reports that vinyasa yoga is one of the most remarkable types of yoga in America. Though some may find this form to be an unchanging series of poses like ashtanga vinyasa, stream vinyasa classes will always be unique experiences, she assures.

Vinyasa yoga styles such as power yoga, Baptiste yoga, Jivamukti and prana stream can be particularly physically and mentally demanding for some students, according to Fleming. These classes can be especially challenging for beginners.

Shala Worsley, a yoga educator at Asheville Yoga Center in Asheville, North Carolina and certified by Yoga Plot, advises that those unfamiliar with vinyasa yoga may find it challenging to keep up with its fast pace. "If you want to try vinyasa but lack some experience," she suggests, "find a studio that offers an adolescent or tired stream class as an option."

Hot Yoga

Samantha Schupp, founder and educator at Healthwise in New York City's hot yoga studio, insists that hot yoga cannot be replicated in a hotter room. According to Samantha, there are distinct styles of hot yoga performed depending on which studio you visit - something guaranteed by Yoga Plot!

Take into Account Every Detail.

While temperature changes in studios can vary (check the class depiction or call the individual studio to pick up on subtleties),

Schupp points out that warming techniques may also differ.

Nearby standard heating, two or three studios use humidifiers to make the space seem hotter. Healthwise recommends infrared power from electric sheets placed on or around the housetop that may feel less restricted than constrained air heat, she notes. The size of the room, climate outside and how busy classes are all factors in determining how bothersome a space feels for students, Schupp adds.

Not All Hot Yoga Classes Are the Same

Hot yoga, also known as "warm yoga," originated during the 1970s with Bikram yoga and eventually power was added to this mix of styles.

Vinyasa yoga or stream-type poses done in a heated studio are commonly referred to as hot yoga. According to Schupp, it would be wise to have some prior yoga experience before participating in such an intensive class;

depending on the studio, an adolescent course might even be offered.

Pregnant Women, People with Heart Conditions and Some Others Should Consult Their MD Before Beginning Hot Yoga Practice

Laskowski emphasizes that yoga generally benefits those in good physical and mental health, regardless of their time commitment. However, those with chronic medical issues, power injuries, heart conditions or who become easily dried out may not be eligible to practice hot yoga, according to Laskowski.

Laskowski recommends consulting your primary care physician prior to undertaking any activity that could place undue strain on your body.

What Are Other Popular Styles of Yoga?

According to Laskowski, there are around 20 basic forms of yoga. He adds that people often have various reasons and goals in mind when seeking out this practice.

Based on your location and the size of the yoga community, you may be able to find these classes nearby. Here is a list of some popular types:

Hatha Yoga

Hatha yoga (pronounced HAH-ta, not - that) encompasses various styles of yoga such as ashtanga, vinyasa and power yoga. Classes tend to be slower-paced than their counterparts in vinyasa classes and may not guarantee progress from one position to the next; presents may be held for several breaths before transitioning onto another position. What remains consistent across various hatha yoga forms is that positions should be related to your breathing models.

Ashtanga Yoga

Ashtanga yoga is an in-the-moment type of practice that moves rapidly from position to position. Rather than stream or vinyasa yoga, there are set sequences which must be performed in a certain order. Ashtanga can be taught either in an educator-driven class setting or through Mysore plan where an educator provides instruction without leading the class; understudies must remember the sequence and timing from memory in this latter case, according to Fleming.

Kundalini Yoga

Kundalini yoga combines positions, breathing, reflection and mantras. Ultimately, this form of practice seeks to "blend" our various energies within us while adding care.

Yin Yoga

Yin yoga is a style of yoga where you stay in one position for an extended period, often on the floor or lying on your back or stomach, according to Fleming. You don't move between poses - instead, you stay rooted in one spot for several minutes at a time.

Chapter 4: Basic Tips Every Yoga Student Should Know

The more you practice yoga, the more positions you'll undoubtedly learn. Everyone starts with a challenging pose but everyone eventually progresses to something similar large. Particular attention should be paid to young adult poses which offer numerous advantages like relieving back tension, expanding hips and creating congruency.

What You May Think of Yoga Mats -- and Other Yoga Props

There's often an unfounded perception that props are only for novices or people with "defects" at yoga, but this couldn't be further from the truth. Both experienced yogis and beginners use props for various reasons, from comfort to making stretches easier or making positions safer if there is a certified issue or block, according to Tune Krokoff - teacher certified by GRYA accredited specialists and Yoga Affiliation as well as author of Yoga

Shines: 108 Direct Practices for Strain Help in 2 Minutes or Less

Krokoff believes props can be a helpful aid in making presents accessible to people of all body types. She notes that those with more lanky arms or an even longer center may require assistance getting into position safely, and suggests using props like blocks or yoga lashes as balancers.

Props can also be an essential element of class, like in seat yoga classes where most of the coordinated poses take place on a seat rather than on the floor, according to Krokoff.

Yoga for Beginners: What You Ought to Be Aware Before Your Five Star Experience

Are you just starting out in yoga and need some tips before heading off on your five star adventure? Props may be just what the doctor ordered!

Are you new to yoga? Make sure you understand these essential points before signing up for a class.

*Observe a class before signing up, according to Judi Bar, yoga expert and program boss at Cleveland Center Success and Preventive Medication who is certified by the Overall Relationship of Yoga Instructors and Yoga Union. If the class seems juvenile, further investigation could be in order. She notes that juvenile classes tend to draw extra young or fit individuals or those with little yoga experience "by and large." To be safe, speak with the educator or watch part or all of the class before committing.

*Try taking a more sedentary class or one designed for children. Make sure the instructor encourages participants to focus on their bodies. "You should feel supported in doing what you enjoy doing on an unpredictable day," according to Bar. Don't even think twice about dropping out of a class that feels like competition if you're just starting out," she adds.

*Conversate with the educator before class begins. Get to know more about them and share with them your most memorable rate, according to Laskowski. "Teachers are more than willing to assist in altering circumstances to ease stressful injuries," he states. "Learners want to hear all of your concerns."

Take the necessary steps to not sweat the small stuff. Remember, everyone was once an adolescent at some point. "Yoga doesn't need to be complicated; no stunning dress or props is required; it should simply be a clear practice," Sherwin explains. "Yoga helps people experience true concordance by then."

Fundamentals of Yoga

Yoga classes consist of many repetitive actions, called poses, along with express breathing systems and reflection standards. If a position causes discomfort or looks too hazardous for an understudy to attempt it, certain modifications or combinations can be made to help students get the most benefit from positions. Props like blocks, covers, lashes -- even seats -- can be utilized to help maximize benefits from positions. Remember: yoga is individual; your best practice depends on individual needs and objectives.

Dr. Roger Cole, Ph.D., a psychobiologic and certified Iyengar yoga educator, notes the numerous advantages to regular yoga practice. Not only does it keep your back and joints in good shape but it can also strengthen muscles while increasing mental clarity, all with the added bonus of relaxation woven into each yoga session by Dr. Cole: "Relaxation is integrated into each yoga meeting."

Dr. Timothy McCall, author of "Yoga as Remedy," states that yoga's focus on breathing can help you find peace within yourself and become more aware of your body; this makes moving much smoother for anyone with any level of mobility issues.

Lately, more evidence is emerging to demonstrate the therapeutic benefits of yoga.

Yoga shows us the many ways it can benefit:
*Decrease back pain: Regular yoga classes offer optional relief from low back discomfort as well as extraordinary, extended get-togethers.

*Support Bones: In a recent study, yoga experts were found to have significantly thicker bone thickness in their spine and hips compared to individuals in a benchmark bundle.

*Cultivate Balance: Male opponents in a lone report demonstrated greater congruency after 10 weeks of yoga classes than they had experienced following an identical benchmark social event with no changes made to their schedules.

*Prevent Mental Debilitation: According to one study, people who did yoga and reflection instead of engaging in cerebral planning exercises performed much better on tests related to visuospatial memory - essential for balance, strategic judgment and the capacity to interpret contradicting information. They were more able to balance their thoughts and make sense of the world.

*Milled Stress: According to an assessment of 72 women, Iyengar yoga reduced mental strain and its related emotional and physiological consequences.

*Relieve misery: In an assessment of coal excavators with chronic obstructive pneumonic sickness (C.O.P.D.), yoga was shown to reduce weakness and tension symptoms.

Yoga Is Ancient, Yet Reigning

Yoga originated with an ancient Indian philosophy. Therefore, many poses associated with the practice have both Sanskrit and English names (for instance, adho mukha svanasana is more often referred to as plunging facing canine pose), making it possible for students to experience both styles of instruction.

No matter if you have ever taken a yoga class, chances are you are familiar with some of its concepts. Have you ever lifted weights? Congratulations - that's yoga.

Coaches and prosperity classes around the globe, along with school and many of today's finest games social events, have begun incorporating yoga into their regular exercises as a means of strengthening mental and physical strength, aiding competitors with improved breathing techniques and increased focus.

Yoga & Assessment

Yoga was long before it became an established physical activity; for much of its history, it served primarily as a form of assessment.

Care with Yoga

In a yoga class, as you explore different methods for doing poses, your instructor may encourage you to pay attention to both your breath and how your body moves during exercises. Unfortunately, they cannot serve as the basis of an effective brain-body connection.

Yoga offers us the unique opportunity to engage all of our body, exploring how different positions affect us. You may notice, for instance, that one side of your body feels different during a stretch than another; or that changing up on one leg helps ease shoulder tension.

Yoga transforms certain activities into tools to aid students with becoming more aware and developing an effective strategy for reflection.

Chapter 5: Finding the Ideal Approach to Consider

Determining an effective strategy for contemplating is important and can be done quickly. We've put together some key pointers that will guide you down a path toward more profound understanding and contentment.

The Breath

Breathing strategies are an integral component of yoga -- not only do they help you stay on track while practicing, but they can also reduce strain, loosen the structure, and quiet your mind.

According to Elena Brower, yoga breathing techniques provide "a gateway into thought," she is the creator of "Speciality of Thought." According to Ms. Brower, more individuals who have recently discovered certified bits of yoga are moving toward contemplation as they recognize that there is an increasing need for space to reflect, release and refocus.

Next we explore breathing systems associated with yoga classes:

Stomach Loosening Up: Also referred to as diaphragmatic or waist breathing, this breathing technique is the most widely practiced in yoga. It encourages clear, competent communication that takes into account all factors.

Try it Out:

1. Inflate your middistrict as you inhale.

2. Exhale deeply to rid yourself of any air that might be present in your abdomen.

Ujjayi or "productive" breath: This kind of deep inhaling allows you to slow and smooth out the rate at which breath comes out. It is often utilized in stream classes to help understudies organize their breathing while they move through positions.

Try it Out:

1. Squeeze the muscles at the back of your throat and inhale and exhale with your mouth closed.

2. To begin, inhale completely and release 33% of the breath, take a moment to breathe out another third, take another moment to relax, exhale the rest of the air you just exhaled - then repeat for several times more.

8. You can then alternate nostril relaxing with exhalation to adjust your sensory system and prepare yourself for contemplation.

Try it: This strategy has been found to be successful at altering sensory perception.

1. Close one nostril and inhale through the open nostril.

2. Exhale through the same nostril.

3. Switch hands and block off one nostril at a time until all 3 have been closed off completely.

4. Inhale through this same nostril and exhale out.

5. Repeat a few times.

Get Your Stuff

Starting a yoga practice doesn't require anything special, but these items may become necessary as you progress.

No Socks, No Shoes - An Issue

Yoga is often done barefoot on a mat. Socks can be hazardous, which is why they are generally discouraged. If you must wear socks while doing yoga, search for sports socks with elastic grasps on the soles.

Yoga Mats

Most yoga studios and exercise centers provide mats; however, many yoga understudies prefer to purchase their own for cleanliness and the variety of material, thickness, and tensile strengths available. You might find that certain kinds of mats work better for you than others depending on what kind of practice you do or if the studio provides specific types of training sessions.

Choose a mat that prevents slips and slides, providing a secure foundation for changing positions quickly. Regularly disinfect your mat with antibacterial wipes; if you plan to rent mats at your studio or exercise center, be sure to bring along some antibacterial wipes in case any need arise.

Garments

Once you select your yoga outfit, any exercise garments should work just fine. However, clothing that is too baggy may cause disruption when progressing into headstand and handstand poses.

Starting a Yoga Practice

To reap the full benefits of yoga, it is important to make it part of your routine daily practice.

Establish a Consistent Yoga Practice

When beginning any new well-being habit, remember that progress takes time. Start small and reasonable; 10 or 15 minutes every day may be more beneficial than attending one class for seven days straight. As the saying goes: "I would much rather have an understudy succeed at doing one minute per day than fail miserably at doing five." Ideally, as you see the benefits of your regular but short practices, chances are good that you will become motivated to do more of them.

Track Down a Class

Yoga can be done from home, but for beginners especially it's recommended to attend at least one or two classes taught by an experienced educator in either private or social settings. Doing this ensures your safety when doing the practices of yoga correctly.

When seeking a yoga educator, look for one with at least 200 hours of teaching certification from an instructor certified with the Yoga Collusion. Such projects should address injury prevention strategies. If you have any specific medical concerns, consult a specialist before beginning to explore which forms of yoga might be most suitable for you.

When looking for yoga studios or rec centers that provide slip-safe mats (if you plan on renting one), and strong, clean blocks for assistance, make sure there is an antibacterial shower or fabrics nearby so you can wipe down your mat after each use.

Need a tight center, strong arms, and defined legs? Grab your yoga mat and prepare to sweat! You'll be amazed at what you can accomplish!

Chapter 6: What Class is Ideal for Me?

Yoga classes come in many varieties today. Some are challenging and will leave you sweating; others are gentle yet supportive. Some educators play music during class; others don't. Some incorporate references to yoga logic or otherworldliness while others don't.

Here are a few types of classes your yoga studio or recreation center might provide:

Hatha: In America today, most yoga styles are hatha yoga - an overall term that refers to the actual act of doing yoga rather than its philosophical significance or philosophical reflections. A Hatha yoga class typically involves stances and breathing activities but it can be hard to tell whether they will be challenging or delicate; inquire with the school or educator for further details regarding classes classified solely as Hatha yoga.

Ashtanga Yoga: This challenging style of yoga is composed of ever-evolving groupings of postures that understudies typically practice on their own with guidance from an instructor. If you think yoga isn't a workout, try an Ashtanga class! Classes often feature high-level poses like arm adjusts and reversals such as headstands or shoulder stands that require expert instruction; amateur students are strongly advised to work with an experienced educator for optimal learning results. Participants in Ashtanga classes tend to retain lessons for yoga reasoning too, making the lessons valuable lifelong!

Power Yoga: Power yoga is a challenging style of yoga aimed at strength-building. These classes may include challenging postures like headstands and handstands that require great stability to complete.

Vinyasa or Stream: Vinyasa classes typically feature an energetic stream of yoga poses that, depending on the level, may include high-level postures like arm adjusts, headstands, shoulder stands, and handstands.

Many vinyasa classes feature music from the teacher's choice as background music.

Iyengar: Are you fascinated by how muscles and joints function together? Then Iyengar yoga is for you. Classes focus on accuracy in postures, with props like covers, blocks, lashes or reinforces to assist students with poses they wouldn't otherwise have the chance to try. Some classes even incorporate ropes that are attached to walls for reversals or different poses; plus they usually incorporate breathing activities as well as references to yoga theory.

Bikram Yoga or Hot Yoga: Looking for an intense workout? Bikram yoga is a set sequence of 26 postures performed in a room warmed to 105 degrees, which some believe allows the muscles to stretch further and accommodate superior cardiovascular exercise. Unlike most yoga classes, Bikram classes always conclude in rooms equipped with mirrors. Hot yoga refers to any warmed room -- typically between 80-100 degrees

Fahrenheit -- where participants engage in heated poses.

Supportive Yoga: If you're searching for a more relaxing approach to your yoga classes, helpful yoga is the perfect choice. This style usually incorporates some relaxing poses that are held for extended periods. Supportive postures include light winds, forward folds and delicate back-twists which may be completed with various props such as covers, blocks or reinforces.

Are you searching for an intense stretching experience? Look no further than Yin Yoga! This form of stretching focuses on strengthening connective tissue around the pelvis, sacrum, spine and knees in order to increase adaptability. Presents usually last three to five minutes in this calm style of yoga that will quickly reveal your capacity for standing still.

It's wise to try out some yoga classes. Your decision on whether or not you take part will depend on whether or not you enjoy the educator, not necessarily how many points it earns.

Class Behavior

Yoga students should be attentive and aware of each other during class. Swarm classes may result in mat-to-mat adjustments, so don't expect much room around you for personal effects. Most yoga homerooms have racks to store your belongings such as keys, drinks, etc. Make sure your cell phone is switched off before entering the studio.

For Bikram or hot yoga classes, bring a towel. You will perspire, and it can help prevent slips.

Classes typically begin with a brief presentation by the educator that highlights one or more topics for the afternoon, such as backbends or specific poses. Afterwards, many instructors will instruct their students to recite "Om" together - an ancient Sanskrit expression signifying the interconnectivity of all things in existence.

No obligation to say "Om": it's your choice whether or not to remain calm during that time.

In yoga classes, some breathing strategies may be intended for clarity while others are not. Understudies must follow their teacher's lead on this matter.

If you need to leave early, notify the educator in advance and try to position yourself near the back of the room so you can leave before unwinding time at the end of class.

A Word to the Over-Achiever: Making a good effort often leads to injury. Staying aware of your actual limitations and when you need to adjust a posture is more beneficial for your body than striving to be the most adaptable or grounded student in class.

Theory

Yoga is a holistic practice, connecting the brain, body and soul.

There are six branches to yoga; each offering its own focus and set of qualities.

These six branches include:

*Hatha Yoga: This physical and mental branch encourages meditation on one's self.

*Raja Yoga: This branch requires serious contemplation as well as strict adherence to eight appendages of yoga - discipline advancements designed for mental clarity.

*Karma Yoga: This approach to management seeks to create a future free from cynicism and childishness.

*Bhakti Yoga: Dedication can take many forms, from positive methods for managing feelings to developing resilience and acknowledgment.

*Jnana yoga: This part of yoga focuses on wisdom, the way of the researcher, and developing knowledge through study.

*Tantra yoga: Tantra represents custom, function or relationship fulfillment.

Chakras can help facilitate these themes.

"Chakra" is an ancient symbol representing a turning wheel. Yoga holds that chakras are central points of energy, thoughts and emotions within our physical bodies; they shape how individuals experience reality through close-to-home responses, desires or revolutions, levels of certainty or dread and even physical side effects and impacts.

When energy becomes blocked in a chakra, it can cause physical, mental or close-to-home irregular characteristics like nervousness, dormancy or unfortunate processing.

Asanas are the physical postures found in Hatha yoga. Yoga practitioners use asanas to release energy and reinvigorate an imbalanced chakra. There are seven major chakras, each with its own special focus:

*Sahasrara: Situated at the crown of your head, the crown chakra represents profound association.

*Ajna: Located between the eyebrows, this third eye chakra represents instinct.

*Vishuddha: The throat chakra represents resistance and verbal correspondence.

*Anahata: The heart chakra, located at the center of the chest, plays an important role in both professional and interpersonal connections. Any imbalances within this chakra will impact oxygen, chemicals, tissue control, and organ management.

*Manipura: Situated in the stomach region, this sun-powered plexus chakra symbolizes fearlessness, intelligence and self-restraint.

*Svadhishthana: Located beneath the stomach button, this sacral chakra symbolizes joy, prosperity and essentiality.

Chapter 7: Ashtanga yoga

Ashtanga yoga draws upon ancient lessons in order to incorporate them into poses and groupings that quickly connect breathing with each development. It became increasingly popular during the 1970s.

Bikram Yoga

People practicing Bikram yoga, also known as hot yoga, typically do so in rooms heated to almost 105oF and 40% relative humidity. It consists of 26 postures followed by two breathing activities.

Hatha yoga

This form of yoga requires people to move through space at a steady rate with little resistance.

Hatha yoga is the traditional term for the physical practice of yoga. Hatha classes often serve as an introduction to the essential poses found within this ancient discipline.

Iyengar Yoga

This kind of yoga practice emphasizes finding the correct alignment in each pose with the help of props like blocks, covers, lashes, seats and supports.

Kripalu Yoga

Kripalu yoga helps practitioners become aware, accept and benefit from their body. An understudy of Kripalu yoga must determine how to find their degree through internal research.

Classes usually commence with breathing exercises and gentle stretches, followed by an array of individual poses before concluding with relaxation and unwinding.

Kundalini yoga

Kundalini yoga is a form of contemplation meant to release stored energy.

Kundalini yoga classes often begin with reciting mantras and conclude with singing. In between, there is emphasis on asana, pranayama, and contemplation that are designed to produce specific results.

Power Yoga

In the late 1980s, professionals created this dynamic and athletic form of yoga within an Ashtanga framework. Sivananda helped popularize it.

This framework utilizes five-point reasoning as its foundation.

This way of thinking aligns with legitimate breathing, unwinding, diet, exercise and positive reasoning as components that together make up a sound yogic lifestyle.

People practicing Sivananda typically start with Sun Salutations and end in Savasana.

Viniyoga

Viniyoga emphasizes structure over capability, breath and variation, redundancy/holding patterns as well as the craft and study of sequencing.

Yin Yoga

Yin yoga emphasizes holding detached models for prolonged periods. This style of yoga works on deep tissues such as tendons, joints, bones and sash (energy fields).

Pre-Birth Yoga

Pre-birth yoga draws upon research to create poses specifically tailored for pregnant women. This style of exercise can help individuals get back in shape after conception, as well as promote overall well-being throughout pregnancy.

Helpful Yoga

This is a relaxing strategy for yoga. One spends four or five basic stances with props like covers and reinforces, allowing the individual to sink into deep unwinding without needing to exert any effort while holding the posture.

Benefits of Yoga

Yoga offers numerous advantages which can help individuals reach their fitness goals.

Survey results show that 94% of adults who practice yoga do so for health benefits.

Yoga offers numerous physical and mental advantages, such as developing muscle fortitude *improving adaptability *facilitating better relaxation *promoting heart wellness*assisting in treating habit formation

*decreasing pressure, tension, melancholy and ongoing suffering

*developing rest and improving general prosperity and personal satisfaction

It would be wise to consult a clinical expert prior to beginning yoga practice for these reasons; dangers and potential side-effects cannot be completely dispelled.

Many forms of yoga are moderately gentle, making them suitable for individuals when a qualified teacher leads the training.

It is rare that doing yoga will result in serious physical issues. The most frequent injuries among yogis include strains and injuries.

Before beginning a yoga practice, individuals might want to consider some potential risks.

Women who are pregnant or have a chronic health issue such as bone misfortune, glaucoma or sciatica should consult with a medical services expert if possible before beginning yoga practice.

Certain individuals may need to modify or avoid certain yoga positions due to their medical condition.

Novices should avoid advanced poses and techniques like Headstand, Lotus Posture, and strong relaxation techniques.

When managing a condition, individuals should never substitute yoga for regular medical advice or put off seeing a healthcare professional about discomfort or other medical problems.

Yoga is an age-old practice that has evolved over time. Nowadays, its focus is more on introspection and physical wellbeing; old yoga didn't place as much emphasis on wellness; rather, it focused on developing mental focus and amplifying profound energy levels.

There is a vast array of yoga styles available. Which type one chooses will depend on their expectations and level of physical readiness.

People with certain ailments, like sciatica, should begin slowly and with caution when exploring this practice.

Yoga can provide a sense of balance and vitality to life. What are the medical advantages of yoga?

Yoga is an ancient practice that emphasizes breathing, strength, flexibility - breathing deep into yourself to develop resilience. Exercising regularly might offer numerous physical as well as psychological wellness advantages like motivating them to practice more *eating more refreshingly *developing their best qualities *reducing feelings of anxiety *inspiring them to reduce alcohol use or smoking

Evidence is mounting that yoga may offer various health benefits. We list these potential advantages below.

Reduces pressure

People often practice yoga to reduce tension and relax. Researchers are currently unraveling the mechanisms of how it does this.

Excessive amounts of synthetic substances like adrenaline or cortisol, which cause acute vein pain and rapid heartbeats, may also contribute to these effects.

Research has demonstrated that people who practice yoga regularly often have low cortisol levels. Furthermore, studies have determined that practicing yoga for approximately 90 days could significantly reduce cortisol and blood pressure while decreasing combustible cytokines responsible for irritation.

Facilitating Anxiety

Most people experience some level of worry from time to time. But anxiety can be caused by many conditions, including caution mix, social strain issues, posttraumatic tension issues (PTSD), and fears.

A 2016 meta-study revealed that practicing Hatha yoga had a beneficial effect on anxiety levels. Notably, those who experienced higher degrees of unease at the start of their assessments found most benefit from practicing yoga.

A more conclusive study from 2010Trusted Source showed that yoga increased mental clarity and anxiety more than walking alone. The researchers suggested this was due to increased amounts of the frontal cortex compound gamma-aminobutyric destructive (GABA).

GABA activity will likely be reduced in those suffering from stress and emotional issues, according to researchers who tested yoga's effect on GABA levels in these individuals.

A recent report explored whether school-based yoga could benefit kids who were feeling stressed. Finding that practicing yoga at the start of each school day for some time further nurtured their wellbeing and wellbeing compared to those practicing it without any guidance or instruction, these results are encouraging.

Critical sorrow affects approximately 17.3 million adults in the U.S. each year, yet yoga has made them all equally effective treatments for distress.

A 2017 groundbreaking study demonstrated the therapeutic effects of yoga on various populations, including people suffering from oppressive disarray, pregnant and postgender women, as well as watchmen.

Research published in 2017 examined people with debilitating conditions that hadn't responded to antidepressants. Concentrated groups who completed two months of Sudarshan Kriya yoga experienced a reduction in troublesome secondary effects, while the control group experienced no improvements.

Experts speculate that yoga could reduce the negative effects of anxiety by decreasing cortisol, or the "stress compound." Thus, experts speculate, yoga might also aid in relieving lower back torment.

Around 80% of adults will experience lower back pain at some point in their lives, which can significantly restrict the ability to perform daily tasks, exercise, and rest. Yoga could be a useful and cost-effective solution for providing relief.

A 2017 study linked yoga practice with lower back relief from discomfort and an improvement in back-related capability.

Chapter 8: Working on Personal Satisfaction during Illness

Many individuals use yoga as part of their regular medical treatment to boost their sense of well-being. There is some evidence to support this notion that yoga could possibly benefit those suffering from certain medical conditions, including:

*Prostate Malignant Growth. Research suggests that participating in yoga two times per week during prostate disease radiation therapy could reduce weakness and enhance sexual and urinary capability.

*Stroke. Yoga may help develop post-stroke balance and engine capability even if someone begins practicing it a half year or more after their stroke.

*Ulcerative Colitis. Regular yoga classes over a prolonged period may help cultivate positive attitudes toward life for those suffering from ulcerative colitis, while also decreasing symptoms and increasing mobility.

*Rheumatoid joint inflammation. A multi-week concentrated yoga course may help alleviate physical and psychological side effects in people suffering from rheumatoid joint pain, as well as reduce aggravation.

Early research into yoga's potential role in increasing personal satisfaction is encouraging. However, more investigations are necessary before analysts can make definitive statements.

The animating cerebrum capability may also provide some benefits.

Studies have suggested that yoga may enhance cognitive functioning and boost energy levels, according to some research studies.

One 2017 review demonstrated that Hatha yoga improved both leadership abilities and personality traits. Leader capabilities are mind exercises related to objective coordinated conduct and controlling profound reactions or tendencies.

Research published in 2012 found that a single yoga session enhanced working memory speed and precision more than one meeting of oxygen-consuming activity. Nonetheless, these effects occurred only after the activity had concluded, and were present moment.

Another investigation suggests yoga may help with mental adaptability, task exchange and data review among older adults.

Preventing coronary illness

Every year in the U.S., around 610,000 people succumb to coronary illness - making it the leading cause of death.

An analysis of yoga and heart health studies revealed that practicing yoga could reduce certain risk factors for coronary illness, such as body mass index (BMI), cholesterol levels, and circulatory strain.

Yoga may help prevent changes to veins that contribute to coronary illness. A study revealed that Bikram yoga, which takes place indoors in a heated room, had beneficial effects on cardiovascular wellness.

Yoga Stances for Amateurs

Start Your Yoga Journey With These Essential Stances

As a new student of yoga, you may feel overwhelmed by all of the stances and their mysterious names. But don't fret; yoga doesn't need to be complex. In fact, if you were just standing there today and extended your arms over your head, that was already doing yoga poses! Furthermore, remember that your practice is an ongoing journey -- giving you plenty of chances to learn many stances along the way.

Many essential yoga stances are instantly recognizable as our bodies twist and overlap into poses. Begin slowly and with mindful breaths by learning some simple yoga poses first - it's wise to keep things straight when just starting out. The models provided here for novices will keep you engaged for some time; then as your training progresses and you gain more experience, more challenging postures may become part of the repertoire.

Remember, you don't have to master each of the 31 poses listed below. They are simply options for you to consider and can be learned at your leisure without any pressure to finish them. Continue reading for more details about each posture.

Sorts of Stances

Find your perfect posture!

Yoga poses differ in accordance with how you move your body to complete them. Here are the essential types of poses commonly practiced:

*Standing Postures: Standing poses are often done first in a yoga class to create heat and get you warmed up. In vinyasa/stream style yoga, these postures may be hung together to form long arrangements; in Hatha classes however, the standing postures might be done exclusively with rests between each one.

*Adjusting Represents: Novice adjustments are an invaluable method for developing the center fortitude necessary for many yoga stances. Though balances may seem challenging at first glance, with regular practice you will begin to improve.

*Backbends: As you develop, your spine will begin to curve more gradually with each successive move, eventually leading to deeper curves. Since backbends are rarely done in daily life, they're essential for spinal health and longevity.1

*Situated Presents: Situated stretches, which typically involve stretching the hips and hamstrings, are often completed near the end of a yoga class once everyone's warm. To make these poses more comfortable, put an expanded cover or block under your seat for added support when doing these stances.

*Resting or Prostratifies: It's essential to become familiar with your resting poses, particularly kid's pose, which you are encouraged to do whenever you need a break during a yoga class. These poses build upon the hip and hamstring work from the situated postures and offer delicate back-bowing, curving, and reversing motions.

Descending Confronting Canine (Adho Mukha Svanasana)

Present Sort: Standing

This posture has long been associated with yoga; however, just because you know about it doesn't make it any less challenging to achieve.

Novices often incline too far forward in this stance, making their feet appear like boards. To maintain balance, keep most of your weight in your legs and come to hip height with heels extending toward the floor (they don't have to touch it).

On the off chance that you have tight hamstrings, bend your knees slightly to accommodate this move. Keep both feet equal.

Mountain Posture (Tad asana)

Present Sort: Standing

Mountain posture may not be as popular as Descending Confronting Canine, yet it is equally significant. This provides us with an ideal opportunity to discuss how your body parts are organized in each position.

Mountain Present creates a straight line from the crown of your head to your heels, with shoulders and pelvis stacked along this line. As each body is different, focus on grounding yourself with your feet while stretching upward with your spine.

Yoga teachers can guide you through this pose in class, reminding you to slide your shoulders down your back and keep weight behind you.

Hero I (Virabhadrasana I)

Present Sort: Standing

In Hero I, it's important to remember that your hips should always face forward. Consider positioning your hips headlights so they are aligned with the front of your mat; this may require taking a more expansive position.

Fighter II (Virabhadrasana II)

Striking this pose from above requires positioning yourself with both legs facing forwards.

Present Sort: Standing

Distinct from Fighter I, Champion II requires the hips and shoulders to open to one side of the mat. As we transition from Fighter I to Champion II, these parts of our bodies become much more mobile.

Turn your back foot so your toes face forward at around 45 degrees angle. In both fighter poses, keep the front knee stacked over the lower leg while keeping your front toes pointed ahead.

Broadened Side Point (Utthita Parvakonasana)

Present Sort: Standing

A Stretched Out Side Point Posture involves carrying your lower arm to your thigh instead of placing it on the floor. Make sure it lays gently on your thigh and doesn't bear too much weight so your shoulders remain open. Alternatively, you could put your hand on a block for extra support.

Before reaching for the floor, consider shifting your center of balance by turning your chest toward the floor instead of toward the roof.

Triangle Posture (Utthita Trikonasana)

Present Sort: Standing

The Triangle can also be changed into an Expanded Side Point by using a yoga block as your base hand if you're uncomfortable bringing your arm down on the floor.

Alternatively, rest your hand higher up on one leg -- such as on your shin or thigh -- but avoid placing it directly onto your knee.

If the posture feels awkward, try twisting both knees inward. This won't look or feel like an articulated curve but rather just enough movement to open your knees and reduce strain on hamstrings.

Triangle training has many benefits: strength (in the legs), adaptability (in the crotch, hamstrings and hips, as well as opening the chest and shoulders), and balance.

Remaining Forward Curve (Uttanasana)

To do this pose, bend forward at the waist, breathe out, and crease over your legs. Assuming the hamstrings feel close from the start, twist the knees so your spine is delivered and let the head hang weighted.

Chapter 9: Switch Fighter (Viparita Virabhadrasana)

Present Sort: Standing

Switch Fighter offers a similar position to Champion I and adds an inviting side curve or optional backbend for added effect.

Maintaining a stable stance requires rooting into the bottom of the front foot, anchoring its external edge on the back foot, and connecting with glutes and hamstrings.

As your gaze climbs toward the palm, keep your front knee following over over your lower leg as you sink further into your hips. This is known as Wreath Posture (Malasana).

Present Sort: Standing

Crouching may not be a natural part of life for many in 21st-century society, but it can be an excellent stretch for muscles around the pelvis - often referred to as a "hip opener" in yoga.

Maybe unsurprisingly, hunching down can actually be beneficial for your feet - which are often neglected. If hunching down is difficult for you, try sitting on a block or moving something under the heels with a towel or cover underneath and press your heels down toward the floor as much as possible.

Half Forward Curve (Ardha Utttanasana)

Present Sort: Standing

This backward twist (also referred to as a "midway lift") is often done as part of the sun greeting grouping and it's expected that your back will arch. But taking time out to ensure your posture remains level can help build body awareness and help with stress relief. Sorting out when your back is level requires effort on your part - something worth investing in for optimal wellbeing.

Looking in the mirror can be useful when starting this pose. You might want to let your hands fall off the ground and onto your legs as high as necessary to keep the back level, and gently twist both knees as needed.

Pyramid Posture (Parsvottanasana)

Present Sort: Standing

Remaining forward twists like Pyramid present are an excellent opportunity to break out your yoga blocks. Place one or both blocks on either side of your front foot so that the floor is raised enough for easy reach of both hands and hamstrings - they will appreciate your thoughtfulness!

Lifted Hands Posture (Urdhva Hastasana)

When performing this pose with lifted hands, consider doing it while standing. Your arms will thank you for it!

Present Sort: Standing

Urdhva Hastasana encourages you to remain grounded with your legs while reaching high with your arms. This full body stretch provides an amazing opening for your yoga meeting.

Low Push

Present Sort: Standing

Your push should begin by creating a right angle with your front leg, so that your knee is straight over your lower leg and your thigh touches the floor. At the same time, keep both hips level and support your back leg with both hands.

Some individuals fail to dive deeply enough into the front leg and hang in the back leg. Check yourself in the mirror to make sure you're doing it correctly.

To adjust, place your hands on blocks as well as lower your back leg onto a mat (with either a wide towel for padding).

Tree Position (Vrksasana) - this pose requires practice!

Present Sort: Standing/Evolving

Tree present is an inconceivable prelude to evolving positions. If you feel yourself starting to become disturbed, don't worry - simply loosen up your hip by moving it slightly sideways on top of your standing leg.

Begin your search on a spot on the floor, and experiment with various foot positions to see which works best for you: Impact can bring up concealment on either your lower leg, on a block, or above or under your knee.

Jumping Toward Canine Split

Present Sort: Standing/Evolving

Demonstrating different positions helps build core strength. In Down Canine Split, focus should be put on how high you can lift your leg by spreading out into two hands and keeping all weight evenly distributed between both of them.

Board Position

Present Type: Evolving

It might seem counterintuitive to refer to the board as "evolving" when there is no chance of falling over, yet that is exactly the focus of what's happening here -- center strength.

Feline Cow Stretch (Chakravakasana)

Present Sort: Backbend

It's the ideal situation: spinal expansion followed by spinal flexion. Moving this way mixes and warms your back, promotes body care, and serves as an introduction to doing vinyasa with coordinated breath enhancements.

Feline Cow might be an essential position to learn when starting yoga, especially if you experience back discomfort. No matter how many classes you attend, keep practicing this stretch in isolation.

Length Position (Setu Bandha Sarvangasana)

Present Sort: Backbend

Length present is an effective system to assess spine expansion, commonly referred to as a backbend. It's relatively effortless to start making progress with this kind of progress since it manages your spine's adaptability and counters the effects of excessive sitting.

If Development gives off an impression of being too silly, try practicing with a block. Try rooting into your feet so you can use your leg muscles for support in this position (Cobra Pose/Bhujangasana).

Present Sort: Backbend

Cobra poses are done periodically throughout the class as part of the vinyasa social event of positions. While a full Cobra with straight arms offers a deep backbend, you can encourage more abdominal strength by doing low Cobras where you lift your chest without squeezing into your hands.

Root into your feet, extend through the crown of the head and expand through your collarbones as you lift the sternum. Tie down your pelvis to the floor before lifting.

Knees, Chest and Facial Design (Ashtanga Namaskara)

Present Sort: Backbend

Ashtanga Namskara was once prescribed to all beginning yoga students as the gateway pose to Chaturanga Dandasana. Unfortunately, its practice has become increasingly problematic over time.

Unprepared students often rush into chaturanga without proper preparation, with its welcoming series for students. Furthermore, planning extra significant backbends requires meticulous consideration and is an impressive endeavor.

Take as much time as necessary and enter the position from a heap-up position. Begin by bringing your knees down onto the mat with your toes tucked under.

At this point, keep your elbows squeezed toward your body as you lower your chest and facial design to the floor. Your shoulders should float over your hands.

Staff Position (Dandasana)

Present Type: Organized

A staff present is distinguished from an organized rendition of the mountain present (above), in that it provides guidelines for creating other organized presents. Partner with your leg muscles and flex your feet for added support.

Lift your chest and relax the shoulders to allow them to hang loosely over your hips. A slight curve in the knees can also help make it easier for your shoulders to stack over your hips.

If you find it difficult to sit straight with your butts level on the floor, try adding a block or two for support. In regular yoga practice, this position prompts an upward reshape - try Shoemaker's Pose (Baddha Konasana).

Present Sort: Organized

Allow gravity to take over when in Shoemaker's position by extending your inside thighs. If this position feels unsafe, props like sitting on a block, pad, or cover can help make this easier by raising your hips so your knees open more easily.

If your knees are high, it takes considerable effort to hold them up and your legs should be allowed to benefit from stretching. A strategy for doing so is placing a block (or something strong and different) under each knee so they have something firm to rest upon.

As it's uncommon to sit this way in ordinary life, this position stretches the excused locale of the body, particularly around the adductor social gatherings of the crotch.

Essential Position (Sukhasana)

Present Sort: Organized

Sitting with fallen legs shouldn't cause concern about being stuck in an uncomfortable situation. Much like Shoemaker's illustration, effective use of props can transform this mess into one that is easy to manage so that the effects of many seats sitting are improved.

Chapter 10: Present Sort: Organized

Turns are an integral part of yoga. They help develop spinal adaptability and can get things moving along in your digestive system (turns can even ease constipation!2).2

It's perfectly acceptable to extend your base leg if it is unusually bowed behind you. Sitting on a cover can also help modify this position, and placing the twisted leg inside of the long leg can be especially helpful when working with shoulder, hip, and spine issues.

Go to Knee Position (Janu Sirsasana) if your base leg feels strangely bent behind.

Present Sort: Organized

Forward turns may be challenging for those with tight hamstrings (i.e., many). Janu Sirsasana provides more freedom since you stretch each leg individually. You could also wrap a lash around your foot to increase reach and flexibility.

Organized Ahead Curve (Paschimottanasana) -

Present Sort: Organized

Hamstrings should always be stretched when beginning yoga exercises. People who sit a lot tend to get tight in these muscles, which can lead to low back discomfort if not stretched properly during organized forward twist. Extending these hamstrings helps alleviate this tension.

This position provides a gentle stretch to the entire back of the body. Twist at your hips, not your midriff, and keep your neck aligned with your spine.

Situated Wide Point Ride (Upavistha Konasana)

Present Sort: Sitting

By opening your legs wide, you can experience an interesting stretch from Paschimottanasana. To do this:

1. Stand with legs spread wide apart.

2. Flex the feet and draw both legs down simultaneously, creating upavistha konasana.

3. Bend your spine forward towards the middle, expanding its curve on inhalations and deepening it on exhalations. This will create a balanced posture.

Though it may appear that the command is to drop your chest to the floor, there's no need to focus on that. Instead, focus on keeping your back level, pivoting your pelvis forward instead of crunching through, and keeping both feet flexed - regardless of how far forward you lean. That said, Blissful Child Posture (Ananda Balasana) should remain unchanged.

Present Type: Recumbent

A contented child is the perfect way to end a yoga session. It also serves as an excellent reminder of the crucial balance that exists between effort and simplicity in yoga.

You should apply some slight tension on your feet to draw them towards your armpits, but not so much that your tailbone takes off the floor. We recommend staying away from drastic measures and instead tracking down the center ground.

Recumbent Spinal Curve (Supta Matsyendrasana)

Present Sort: Recumbent

An inactive curve is an ideal way to end a yoga class, though there's nothing stopping you from trying this pose at the start of your training regimen. Ultimately, the placement of your legs depends entirely on individual preference.

You have two options for twisting: either fix the top leg and grab your foot, or curve them around each other (as in Hawk pose) to extend external hips. Keep knees following midriff.

Youngster's Posture (Balasana)

Present Sort: Resting

Your child's posture during yoga class is critical; if you ever feel exhausted, don't assume the educator will require a break.

Instead, try your best to relax into whatever position feels most natural for them.

Start by moving into Youngster's pose and rejoin the class when you feel ready. This posture provides a gentle stretch to your back, hips, thighs and lower legs without taxing strength or stability.

Youngster's Pose offers the ideal example of yoga: being open to your body's signals and prioritizing them over any external influences.

Carcass Posture (Savasana) allows for this kind of insight.

Present Form: Resting

Many yoga sessions end with you lying level on your back in Body Present. This is the basic progression between the end of your practice and everyday life; carrying the body to quietness triggers the brain to keep up with it - which may prove challenging at first but becomes easier with training and instruction.

Step-by-step instructions for beginning yoga can help make this transition smoother for you.

Yoga has often been seen as a safe activity, particularly when practiced under the guidance of an accredited teacher. Although experiencing severe injuries while practicing yoga is rare, some individuals do experience injuries and strains while partaking in this form of physical fitness.

Yoga offers a range of styles, from the relaxing to the energetic. Popular types include: *Hatha yoga* *Vinyasa yoga

*Bikram Yoga

*Ashtanga yoga

*Iyengar yoga

*supportive yoga.

When starting yoga, individuals might want to join a beginner's class with an educator who can demonstrate the appropriate postures and methods.

Learning from online recordings or applications could lead to incorrectly configured poses that could cause injury in the long run.

Here is a rundown of some common yoga mistakes:

Overall, yoga is a safe way to increase physical activity and might also have numerous medical advantages. According to studies, it may: *decrease pressure* *ease tension* assist with managing discouragement* decrease lower back torment

*Support those suffering from persistent circumstances or intense illnesses by offering personal satisfaction programs *Energizing mind capability

**Help prevent coronary illness

Lastly, try yoga as an interesting hobby - join a class taught by a certified educator to keep away from wounds

Never substitute specialist-recommended clinical treatment with alternative or complimentary methods.

Chair Yoga

Chair yoga is a delicate practice wherein poses are performed while sitting or with the assistance of a chair. Seat yoga classes cater to those with physical limitations or seniors who find regular yoga meetings too challenging, making it an ideal option for beginners or anyone wanting an easygoing approach to their practice.

Seat yoga may be integrated into a standard Hatha yoga class to assist those with balance issues or any individual who has difficulty getting down onto and off of the floor.

Seat yoga is similar to regular yoga in that it builds adaptability, strength, and body mindfulness. Standing postures are used as the starting point for this form of practice while the seat helps with balance development. In addition, Seat yoga may include pranyama breathing procedures as well as reflection for improved concentration, mental clarity, and relaxation.

Seat yoga allows for many variations on standard yoga poses, such as backbends, turns, hip openers and forward folds. For instance, in a seat mountain pose the yogi sits with their feet level on the floor and their knees at 90-degree angles. Their arms are then raised towards the sky with palms facing upwards; this basic pose can either be performed while sitting or using a handle on the rear of the seat for support.

In Times of Stress and Vulnerability, Your Doshas Might Feel Empty.

To help identify which dosha is dominant, we created the accompanying test to identify it.

For those of us born in the '90s, Mary Ann Wilson's "Sit and Be Fit" and subsequent episodes of "Sesame Road" on PBS taught us that you don't need to get up from your seat in order to have fun. If there's one lesson

Mary Ann Wilson taught us, it's that being dynamic doesn't need to take you away from where you sit.

Seat yoga is an ideal way to get going without needing to get up - neon sweat groups are optional. It's the ideal choice if you need extra assistance during your yoga practice and it can even add some streamlining into your work-from-home daily schedule.

Chapter 11: What exactly is Chair Yoga, exactly?

Chair yoga enables individuals to experience yoga poses while sitting. By adding the support of a seat, these benefits become accessible for more individuals regardless of age, adaptability level, wounds or portability issues.

Even while sitting, you can do various winds, twists, and stretches from Feline Cow to Urdhva Hastasana. Experiment with seat yoga by trying these moves!

Why practice seat yoga?

Much like other forms of yoga, seat yoga has numerous medical benefits that are accessible to anyone who wants it. Here are a few scientifically supported reasons why:

*Strongerness, Perseverance and Adaptability. According to a recent report, scientists concluded that a 12-week Hatha yoga program improved members' solidarity, perseverance and adaptability.

*Mental Clarity. Yoga has long been known to promote mental clarity. A 2019 survey of 11 examinations suggested that yoga may further develop certain cerebrum structures and may help stave off age-related declines in mind capacity.

*Balance. For older adults, falls can be a serious concern. In 2012, researchers examined the experiences of more mature individuals who had recently suffered falls and discovered that seat yoga helped to promote flexibility and equilibrium.

*Torment and exhaustion can help. In a 2018 study of older adults with osteoarthritis, those who led yoga for an extended period showed greater reductions in torment and weakness than their non-yoga conditioned peers.

*Stress Reducing. A 2016 study discovered that an ordinary yoga practice decreased cortisol (the key pressure chemical) levels in individuals suffering from anxiety or distress.

Seat yoga enables individuals to perform certain poses while sitting, making the poses accessible and beneficial to all. Like traditional yoga, seat yoga has numerous benefits such as decreasing pressure and improving one's solidarity, adaptability and equilibrium.

People with portability issues or wounds, in particular, will find this exercise especially beneficial. Make sure to visit with your doctor first for further instructions and security - you deserve it!

Seat Yoga Benefits Everyone

Key Points to Remember about Seat Yoga for Every Age and Body

Important reminders.

*Seat yoga allows you to perform poses while sitting or using a seat for balance.

This form of practice offers many similar advantages as traditional yoga, such as building strength, adapting abilities and mental wellbeing.

*This training is ideal for more seasoned adults, those with specific ailments, and those who work at a desk every day.

Yoga offers numerous benefits, from pain relief to greater adaptability. No wonder then that over 90% of Americans practice it for their wellbeing and health. But for some individuals - especially those with restricted flexibility or ongoing conditions like joint pain or coronary illness - practicing traditional yoga may prove challenging.

Luckily, seat yoga could be an alternative solution. It incorporates situated poses which make the training more accessible. Read on to become familiar with seat yoga, including key postures to begin your practice.

Altered seat yoga utilizes many of the same muscles as traditional yoga stances, providing it with similar medical benefits. Exercising seat yoga regularly can:

Enhance Equilibrium and Adaptability

Maintaining equilibrium and adaptability are essential for overall well-being and prosperity. Not only does it reduce your risk of injury, but it can also help you remain independent as you age. It is no surprise that 3 million more mature adults visit trauma centers regularly for fall-related wounds. A recent report revealed that seniors in a retirement community had been practicing yoga two or three times per week for some time. At the end of the review, participants completed most postures while sitting or standing and using a seat for balance. By the end of it all, members could benefit from improved body adaptability and static equilibrium, reduced anxiety toward falling, and greater trust in their own abilities.

Further, customary yoga may help individuals build muscle tone and strength. A 2021 survey found that seat yoga helped more mature adults maintain muscle strength as they aged, as research suggested. Furthermore, scientists noted that seat-based practice had an impact on upper-and lower-body capability - particularly important given that bulk declines with age as well as a potential lack of social support systems among senior citizens.

Benefit Your State of Mind and Mental Prosperity

Rehearsing yoga may provide emotional benefits like less nervousness and an improved disposition. Research has suggested these effects are common across various styles of yoga, including seat yoga. In one limited scale review, more mature adults took seat yoga classes one time per week for three months; after those same individuals reported improvements such as less pressure, improved temperament, fewer fits of anxiety; they also saw improvements in their general wellbeing, physical capability, and social prosperity.

Support with managing persistent circumstances

Situated yoga may offer assistance to individuals managing ongoing medical conditions like Type 2 diabetes. A recent pilot study looked into the effects of a 10-minute seat yoga program on those living with diabetes; members received standard care and were encouraged to incorporate daily practice into their day-to-day lives. After three months, results showed improvements in glucose, pulse, and circulatory strain levels.

Diminish Ongoing Anger

About 20% of adults suffer from persistent agony that can interfere with daily activities. But research is showing that yoga may be a successful solution for these individuals; one review suggested practicing chair yoga might help older individuals reduce pain and weakness caused by osteoarthritis.

Who Should Try Chair Yoga?

Seat yoga can be enjoyed by all, but its adjusted practice might be especially beneficial for certain groups such as:

*Individuals 65 and older: Chair yoga can be a beneficial practice for mature adults due to its protected atmosphere, low-impact nature, reduced risk of falls and portability. Consequently, this age group may find more interest in chair yoga.

*Individuals with ongoing medical issues: Studies are showing that yoga may provide assistance to individuals managing chronic illnesses (and related pain) such as joint inflammation, diabetes, and dementia.

* Individuals with Limited Mobility: Situated yoga provides the benefits of traditional yoga to individuals with mobility issues. Seat yoga has been shown to benefit those suffering from various sclerosis and recovering from spinal line wounds.

Individuals working in an office: Sitting for extended periods of time can cause depletion, hypertension and torment to the lower back, neck, and shoulders. Rehearsing yoga at work might alleviate back discomfort while improving mental wellbeing; one investigation found that only 15 minutes of seat yoga per day can improve physical and psychological pressure levels.

Prior to beginning seat yoga, it's wise to consult your medical services provider if you have any health concerns or conditions.

How Often Should You Practice Chair Yoga?

There is no set rule when it comes to practicing chair yoga. However, the Centers for Disease Control and Prevention suggest that adults 65 or older get two days of reinforcing activities and three days of equilibrium exercises each week. So starting with some sessions of chair yoga several times each week could be a good place to start.

No matter what, remember that any activity is better than none. Research has even indicated that even occasional yoga meetings could benefit more mature adults.

Chair Yoga: Accessible, Delicate and Amazing for Every Body

Are you having flexibility or equilibrium issues or simply seeking a gentle way of practicing yoga, seat yoga poses may be just what the doctor ordered! Seat yoga has many benefits for those with more physical challenges as well as providing some gentle yet challenging workouts. In this article I'll provide more information about what seat yoga is, its advantages and potential risks as well as provide some authentic seat yoga postures to get you started with this amazing form of therapy.

Seat yoga is a delicate form of yoga, and similar to other varieties it has several benefits: *Better developed strength, equilibrium and adaptability

*Decreased pressure

*Enhanced concentration mindfulness and certainty

*Less actual torment

Chair Yoga Contraindications

While seat yoga offers many benefits, there are still a few contraindications or restrictions that could prevent you from engaging in this practice. If you're uncertain whether it is safe for you to begin or continue doing seat yoga, consult your doctor first. These include ongoing cardiovascular failure or customary chest torments as examples of why not.

*Intense Disease

If you have hypertension, coronary illness, joint inflammation or issues, or have had a hip substitution done, contact your primary care physician for their endorsement and guidance.

Five Benefits of Chair Yoga and Five Poses to Get Things Moving

Yoga has been shown to improve general wellbeing when practiced regularly. Like many types of activity, it should be adjusted for individuals of varying capacities. Seat yoga is one such delicate form that can be done sitting on a seat or remaining on the ground with assistance from a seat. Some benefits of seat yoga include greater adaptability *better fixation *expanded strength *lift your mindset *minimized pressure and joint strain

Chair Yoga Positions for Home Practice

Seat yoga refers to a collection of practices that adapt traditional yoga poses so they can be performed from a chair. These modifications make yoga accessible1 to those who have difficulty standing, lack the mobility to move fully from sitting positions to prostrate ones, or need an occasional break from office tasks.

Repetition of key body mechanics from single positions occurs as before. While sitting, understudies can do various turns, hip stretches, forward turns and delicate backbends.

Chapter 12: Who Can Arrange Yoga Classes?

Seat yoga can be tailored to accommodate anyone who desires to participate in the gradual expansions of yoga and may (or may not) have accessibility barriers. For instance, seat yoga is accessible for those who require extra assistance, are dealing with a major issue, or require an organized approach when planning their activities.

Seat yoga classes are increasingly common in senior living facilities and retirement relationships, as extra-retired adults are its biggest supporters. However, individuals who are obese or have neurological diseases6 may find difficulty accessing these large doorways for seat yoga. Office workers could also benefit when mixing seat yoga with other activities to keep things moving smoothly.

When It Comes to Yoga Seats

Since seat yoga is all about adaptability, don't feel bad if the seat you use isn't huge; other seats will do just as well. Wheeled seats tend to be unsteady and should be avoided; otherwise, most other options should suffice. If space is tighter than expected, try placing blocks or a thin yoga mat underneath your feet for extra support and stability.

Five Seat Yoga Poses You Can Do Anywhere

Yoga can be done wherever there's a seat available. Here are some popular focal seat positions (called asanas) to get you started on your yoga journey. These poses are incredibly adaptable, allowing for easy transitions into working out while doing other things.

Seated cat cow | Working from Home

When working from home or anywhere else, these poses offer tremendous flexibility to adjust according to work demands or other commitments.

Begin by placing your hands on your thighs and sitting up tall. As you exhale, round your back, pull in your abs, tucking the tailbone under and bring your jaw into your chest. Be as round in the upper back as possible while pushing your mid-back toward the seat - this is known as feline posture.

As you breathe in, allow your paunch to push ahead, curve back, send the sternum forward and turn upward toward the roof (if your neck is agreeable), or keep your head lined up with the floor as if there's a cow present.

Replay this movement several times, breathing in as a feline and out as a cow.

Seated cat cow

Start by placing your left hand on your right knee and placing your right arm over the rear of your seat. Take four deep breaths in, exploring your right shoulder as you inhale. As your spine protracts on each inhale, experience an even deeper bend on the exhale. Exhale back to focus and repeat on the opposite side.

Seated Chest Opener

Sit on the edge of your seat and place both hands behind your back. As you breathe in, raise both hands far up into the clouds from behind while tenderly lifting your jaw away from your chest. As you exhale, bring down both hands back down.

Repeat this movement twice on each breath. Alter the hold of your hands and rehash.

Seat pigeon/hip opener

Place your right lower leg on top of your left knee, allowing it to unwind out to one side while keeping your foot flexed. As you breathe in, sit up tall and enjoy this stretch. To deepen it even more, put your hand on top of that same knee and apply gentle tension with it. Alternatively, keep your back level while twisting protracted and beginning to tip forward from your hips for even greater release.

Remain for three to five breaths and repeat on the opposite side.

Seat forward fold:

Start with your hands on top of your thighs and take a deep breath in. As you exhale, draw in at your hips instead of raising the upper back, hanging your body over your legs with one arm holding each elbow as they hang toward the floor. Let your head and neck hang weighty over as you let go on each breath; on exhaling back in, let those hands lie back on top of your thighs before gradually rolling back up again to where you started.

Chair Cat-Cow Stretch

Sit on a seat with your spine long and two feet planted firmly on the floor. Place your hands kneeling or at your highest points of your thighs.

With each breath in, curve your spine and roll your shoulders down and backward, bringing them onto your back in what we refer to as "the cow position".

On a breath out, round your spine and lower your jawline to your chest; this is known as the feline position.

Continue breathing inwardly into a cow pose while exhaling into feline for five breaths.

Chair Raised Hands Pose - Urdhva Hastasana

On an inward breath, raise your arms toward the roof.

Maintain a great chest area posture with shoulders relaxed and ribs confined, sitting normally over your hips. Secure your sit bones in place in your seat and reach up from there.

Chair Forward Bend - Uttanasana

On an exhalation, take a forward twist around the legs. Allow the hands to fall onto the floor if they reach it; let your head hang weighted.

On an inward breath, raise the arms back up over your head. Repeat this movement several times with each breath.

Chair Extended Side Angle - Utthita Parsvakonasana

After your last forward twist, remain collapsed. Bring the passed-on fingertips to the floor outwardly from your left foot. If your left-hand doesn't come down smoothly on its own, place a block underneath it or carry it on one knee and turn from that point.

On a breath in, open your chest and curve to one side by raising your right arm and looking up at the roof. This is your seat rendition of broadened side point present. Hold here for several breaths before bringing that arm back down on an exhale.

Do this same pose with your right arm down and left arm up.

Chair Pigeon - Eka Pada Rajakapotasana

Return to sitting. Bring your right lower leg over and place it near your left thigh, keeping the knee following wherever possible. Maintain this seat pigeon position for three to five breaths.

You could continue the curve to deepen the stretch if desired. Return with the left leg.

Chair Eagle - Garudasana

Assume a falcon is present and place your right thigh over your left thigh. Fold the right foot as far over as possible over the left calf, and cross both arms at the elbow. Twist both arms together before carrying both palms towards contact.

Lift the elbows while dropping the shoulders away from your ears. Hold for three to five breaths.

Repeat on the opposite side.

Chair Spinal Twist - Ardha Matsyendrasana.

Come to sit sideways on the seat, looking to one side. Curve your middle toward the left while clutching the rear of the seat for a spinal turn.

Retract your spine on each breath in and turn it out with each exhale for five breaths.

Move your legs over to the right half of the seat and rehash the curve on that side.

Chair Warrior I - Virabhadrasana I

Maintain balance by lifting one leg over and swinging it away while simultaneously supporting your other leg.

Place the left foot on the floor, generally lined up with the seat of the chair and fix its position.

Keep your middle looking over towards the right leg as you raise both arms to the roof on each exhale from Chair Warrior II - Virabhadrasana II. Hold for three breaths.

Chair Warrior II - Virabhadrasana II

On an exhale out, open up the arms with the right arm drawing nearer and the left returning.

Step the passed-on hip back and turn away so it aligns with the front of the seat.

Glance out over right fingertips and hold legend II for three breaths.

Reverse Warrior

Allow the given arm to plunge the left leg and lift the right arm up towards the rooftop on a take-in for pivot legend. Hold for three breaths.

Bring both legs up towards the front of the seat before shifting your position sideways on it facing left and performing three hero stances on that side.

Finally, Enjoy This Relaxation Moment with Chair Savasana

Take two to three minutes to sit quietly with your eyes closed and place your lap near the end of your preparation. This arranged savasana will help your body rest from all of the positions you have just done, allowing you to move into other parts of your day more easily.

Chapter 13: Ujjayi Breathing

Begin with a new beginning: Sit up tall at the edge of your seat and place both hands on your midsection. Inhale deeply through your nose, stretching out through sides and midriff, before exhaling comfortably. Repeat this process for ten breaths.

Cat/cow

Take a deep breath in and bend your back to look toward the rooftop. Inhale out through your spine, pulling in your abs and changing your posture. Repeat this exercise multiple times for relief from back and neck strain.

Circles

Without moving your chest area, circle your hips clockwise several times and then counterclockwise several times to stretch and relax the hip muscles.

Sun Invite Arms

Sitting tall, take in and lift your arms with palms facing upwards. On an exhale out, float them back down towards your sides a few times for extra flexion in your spine as well as strain in shoulders and neck.

Sun Invite With Turns

Stand tall while taking in and lifting arms above yourself with hands clasped together.

Repeat the previous action, adding a turn as you inhale. Do this on both sides separately, holding each curve for five seconds.

High Extraordinary Ventured Region Side Slopes

For a significant spine and shoulder stretch, lift your arms and weave them together before you. Then turn them towards the rooftop as you fix your arms over your head. Cover this suitable for three breaths, then relax for three.

Hawk Arms

To eliminate any shoulder tension, try this move: extend your arms out to each side and then bring one under the other before reaching shoulder level. While bowing your arms at the elbows, drive yourself so your palms meet at shoulder level and hold for five breaths before relaxing and repeat with the opposite arm on top.

Helped Neck Stretches

FYI: Our necks often experience significant strain. To reduce this, take your right arm and fold it around your head until your palm faces your left ear. Allow your head to drop to that shoulder, hold for five breaths, then switch sides by running against the norm side.

Lower Leg to Knee

The hip area can be a major source of tension. To relax, sit upstanding, contort your right knee, then place the right lower leg over your left knee. For an even deeper stretch, slant forward for added benefit; hold for five breaths then alternate sides.

Goddess with a Turn

Try this incredible hip stretch: Extend your legs wide and curve your foot out. Place your right arm inside of your right leg, coming toward the floor. Lift your left arm toward the rooftop and bring in your look into your left side palm. Hold for five breaths then alternate on this side intermittently.

Legend 2

Here's an effective technique to develop sureness and get a full-body stretch at once. Sit tall at the edge of your seat, turn your right knee outward, stretch out your disregarded leg behind you, then push down through your outside heel. Hold for five breaths before alternately going against the norm side.

Forward Overlay

End your meditation by taking a calming forward curve, which allows blood to stream to your brain. Sit tall and straight in a chair. Wrinkle over your legs so that your head, neck, and body hang limp. Hold for however long desired before returning to a sitting position.

Yoga Can Cut Into Your Prosperity

My experience inspired me to examine the many assessments of yoga both in India and the West to see how it could both prevent sickness and aid with recovery from it. What I observed was that:

Increases flexibility

Yoga offers the greatest versatility of all, and that is perhaps its primary advantage. When doing five-star exercises, chances are you won't even have the option to touch your toes let alone do a backbend! However, if you stick with it, you will experience consistent delivery and eventually, seemingly unattainable stances will become possible. Furthermore, you might notice that a seemingly overwhelming difficulty starts to fade away - this is no random event! Tight hips can place undue strain on the knee joint due to an improper alignment of the thigh and shinbones. Tight hamstrings may lead to an alteration in the lumbar spine, causing backache. Furthermore, muscle and connective tissue adhesion from belts or ligaments may create a sad position.

Muscle determination creates muscle growth.

Strong muscles do more than just make us look amazing; they protect us from conditions like joint pain and back discomfort, helping to prevent falls for older individuals. Furthermore, when you develop strength through yoga, it balances out with flexibility; if you just went to the acting neighborhood lifting loads without stretching first, coarseness could develop leading to an impediment to adaptability.

What's going on

Your head is like a bowling ball -- huge, round, and crucial. When placed straight over an upright spine, it requires much less effort from your neck and back muscles to support itself. However, pushing it too far ahead can put undue strain on those muscles. Holding that forward-slanting ball for eight or 12 hours a day doesn't come as any huge shock when your energy reserves are depleted. Weariness will likely not be your top concern either. Hanging from this position has been known to cause back, neck, and other muscle and joint issues; over time your body could compensate by fixing everything in your neck and lower back which could cause pain and degenerative joint wretchedness of the spine.

Thwarting Tendon and Joint Breakdown

Yoga exposes your joints to their full range of movement, helping prevent degenerative joint aggravation or diminish lack by "squeezing and soaking" areas that don't get used frequently. After all, the tendon is like a sponge; it gets new updates right when its fluid is squeezed out and another stock can be held. Without sensible food though, that exonerated region could eventually wear away, revealing bone-like segregated brake pads underneath.

Shields Your Spine

Spinal circles - those protective discs between vertebrae that can herniate or pack nerves - need regular strengthening. That is how they get their upgrades. By practicing consistent asana with plenty of backbends, forward bends, and winds in your practice, you'll help keep those plates smooth. Yoga's great length versatility is well known but especially important for spinal health.

Increases Bone Prosperity

Yoga not only enhances bone prosperity but it improves bone prosperity as well.

Weight bearing movements such as yoga can strengthen bones and prevent osteoporosis. Some poses, like Adho Mukha Svanasana (Plunging Defying Canine) and Urdhva Mukha Svanasana (Up Standing up to Canine), even help build up arm bones which are particularly vulnerable to breakages due to osteoporosis. An unpublished audit conducted at California State School in Los

Angeles revealed that yoga practice increased vertebral thickness through reduced levels of cortisol--possibly due to its capacity for decreasing cortisol--also helping maintain calcium within those same bones.

Yoga improves circulation

Yoga not only gets your blood flowing, but the stretching stretches you learn in yoga can help loosen up tight spots like grip and feet. Furthermore, yoga adds more oxygen to cells - improving their capacity to perform their duties better. Bending positions are carefully designed to draw out venous blood from inside organs and allow oxygenated blood to enter after the twist is applied. Modified poses such as Headstand, Adho Mukha Vrksasana (Handstand), and Shoulder Stand encourage venous blood from the legs and pelvis to flow back towards the heart, where it will be oxygenated before entering into your lungs for renewal. Yoga may help alleviate symptoms associated with heart or kidney issues by encouraging you to extend your legs. Furthermore, yoga boosts levels of hemoglobin and red platelets - oxygen carriers for tissues - which further contributes to relaxation. Additionally, aspirin thins the blood by making platelets less flavorless and decreasing group-propelling proteins in it. This could potentially prevent respiratory disappointments and strokes since blood bunches are often responsible for these fatal incidents.

Chapter 14: Channelling Your Lymph and Lifting Invulnerability

By understanding and stretching muscles, moving organs around, and coming all through yoga positions, you increase the misuse of lymph (a gooey fluid rich in safe cells). This aids the lymphatic structure to fight defilement, destroy destructive cells, and dispose of harmful material caused by cell working.

Increases Your Heart Rate

Doing yoga also has been known to increase heart rate since it helps increase oxygenation to cells while decreasing anxiety levels.

By regularly increasing your heartbeat into oxygen-depleting range, you reduce the likelihood of having a coronary episode and can provide comfort in times of despair. Yoga may or may not have a meditative effect, but those who practice regularly or take Ashtanga classes can find that even moderate yoga increases your heartbeat to an oxygen-intense level. Even gentle yoga practices that don't elevate the pulse that much can still benefit your cardiovascular health. Studies have demonstrated that yoga practice reduces resting heart rate, increases diligence and can diminish exercise-induced high-influence impressions. One such test revealed subjects taught only pranayama could do more action with less oxygen intake.

Drops Your Circulatory Strain

If you have hypertension, yoga could be beneficial. According to two studies published in The Lancet, people with hypertension experienced benefits from Savasana (Corpse Stance) by lying on an affection seat after three months. After that time had elapsed, Savasana was linked with a 26-point drop in systolic heartbeat (the top number) and 15 points drop in diastolic circulatory strain (the base number); the higher the initial heartbeat, the greater the drop). Additionally, deals with adrenal organs

Yoga has the potential to reduce cortisol levels. But why? Traditionally, adrenal glands will release cortisol during times of acute crisis to maintain safe capacity. Cortisol levels that remain elevated even after a crisis can wreak havoc on your mental structure. Brief increases in cortisol may aid with long-term memory, but sustained high concentrations may harm memory and lead to significant changes to the frontal cortex. Additionally, excessive cortisol has been linked to critical depression, osteoporosis (the loss of calcium and other minerals from bones that prevents new bone formation), hypertension, and insulin resistance. Rodents with high cortisol levels often exhibit "food-chasing behavior"-- the urge to consume extra calories when distressed, distressed, or pushed. As a result, rodents become overweight and their risk for diabetes and coronary episodes increases.

Feeling hopeless? Try Lotus. More impressively, take up a backbend or move into Ruler Craftsman Stance for some added relaxation and invigoration. An analysis conducted at the School of Wisconsin revealed that an anticipated yoga practice also produced feelings of gloom while increasing serotonin levels and decreasing monoamine oxidase (a protein which isolates neurotransmitters and cortisol). Richard Davidson Ph.D. found that meditators' left prefrontal cortex showed greater development when practicing mindfulness - likely leading to additional joy and improved safety abilities as well. Long stretch specialists showed even greater excitement on their left sides than other practitioners did.

Lays the Foundation for a Health Lifestyle

Move more, eat less -- that is the motto of many well-being food nuts. Yoga can help with both of these goals by getting you moving and burning calories while strengthening relationships with divine and near and dear elements in your life that could potentially hinder progress with eating or weight issues. Yoga also gives you energy to become a more mindful eater, further cultivating its benefits throughout various aspects of your life. One major advantage of practicing yoga is how its practices resonate throughout various areas of your life.

Cuts Down Glycemia

Yoga has been found to decrease glucose and LDL ("terrible") cholesterol while raising HDL ("extraordinary") cholesterol. Diabetes patients have seen benefits in multiple ways from yoga: by decreasing cortisol and adrenaline levels, encouraging weight loss, and suppressing insulin effects. With lower glucose levels comes less of a chance for diabetic disarray such as coronary episodes, kidney disillusionment or visual inadequacy; getting your levels under control reduces these risks significantly.

Additionally it assists with focus - helping focus!

Yoga emphasizes being in the present. Studies have demonstrated that standard yoga practice enhances coordination, reaction time, memory and even insight levels. People who practice Powerful Reflection show greater ability to deal with issues as well as security and audit information better - likely because their perspectives are less redirected by repetitive loops of thought.

Relaxes Your Development

Yoga encourages you to slow down, take a deep breath, and focus on the present by shifting from the sympathetic nervous system (or diligence response) to parasympathetic material construction. With this last option, Herbert Benson M.D. helps quiet power regions for relaxation; reduce breath and heartbeat rates; decrease circulatory strain; add nourishment to digestion bundles and regenerative organs with his "Jump Around Town" reaction.

Work on Your Concordance

Yoga not only improves proprioception (the capacity to detect body movement and location) but it also promotes balance. Individuals with abnormal poses or defective improvement plans tend to have poor proprioception, leading to knee issues and back discomfort. Improved equilibrium could mean fewer falls for some; some devotees even go so far as to enter an extra entryway and then surrender admission into nursing homes or never enter at all. As we near the end of our lives, positions like tree pose can help us feel less unequal both on and off the mat.

Remain Aware of Your Material Construction

Yoga offers some extraordinary powers to those at its most basic levels. Some practitioners have been known to set off exceptional heart rhythms, create vivid idea wave models and even raise the temperature of their hands by 15 degrees Fahrenheit using mental imagery. If these yogis can do that with yoga, maybe there's another way to manage this stress besides encouraging your pelvis to endure only during periods when trying for pregnancy or quickly unwind while dealing with insomnia.

Release Stress in Your Person

131

Have you ever found yourself stopping, shifting the steering wheel, or distorting your face as you stare into a computer screen? Does this release tension in your life? These tendencies can cause mild to moderate pressure, muscle weariness and facial disturbance in your wrists, arms, shoulders, neck and face; which in turn may extend and negatively impact your demeanor. At some point during yoga practice, you will likely notice where there are tensions: Your tongue, eyes, or muscles in front of and behind you could all benefit from some attention. By tuning in and paying attention, these areas could benefit from some choice to move some strain away. As for other recognizable muscles like quadriceps, trapezius and gluteus maximus; basic stretching activities could help find a satisfactory way to relax them.

Upholds you as you keep on recovering

Chapter 15: Helps Maintain the Value of Your Protected Casing

Asana and pranayama work on the safe limit, but reflection has revealed that they provide the most profound benefit here. They appear to support and strengthen the safe structure when needed (like raising vaccination steps prior to an immunization) or reduce it when needed (like moderating an inadequately solid sure capacity in conditions like psoriasis).

Yogis often take deeper breaths at a slower rate, giving their lungs space to breathe freely. A recent report published in The Lancet revealed that yoga's "complete unwinding" procedure helped those suffering from lung issues due to congestive cardiovascular breakdown improve their breathing patterns. After one month, their average resting respiratory rate dropped from 13.4 breaths per second down to 7.6, their movement limit significantly expanded and oxygen content of their blood increased too.

Furthermore, yoga has been known to treat various ailments.

Facilitates Your Anger

Yoga has the potential to reduce stress. Studies have found that asana, meditation or a combination of both have been known to decrease discomfort in individuals suffering from joint pain, back pain, fibromyalgia, carpal passage disorder and other persistent circumstances. When your stress is alleviated your mindset improves; you become more energetic and require less medication for daily tasks - leading to less need for medications overall.

Gives You Inward Strength

Yoga offers inward strength which can be utilized towards alleviating mental fatigue

Yoga can help you make changes in your everyday life, which may be its greatest asset. Tapa, the Sanskrit word for "heat," is what drives yoga practice and creates the discipline needed for successful completion. With just a little effort you may start eating better, exercising more or finally giving up smoking after years of unsuccessful attempts!

Interfaces you with direction

A great yoga instructor can do wonders for your wellbeing. Uncommon ones go beyond simply leading you through postures; they offer invaluable advice, measure when to push harder in poses or back off, provide hard truths with compassion, help you relax, upgrade and customize your training program - a deferential relationship is invaluable in this pursuit of betterment. A trusting relationship with an instructor goes a long way toward improving overall wellbeing.

Helps Keep You Calm

If your medication cabinet appears to be running out of space, yoga may be worth trying. Studies of individuals with asthma, hypertension, Type II diabetes and fanatical impulsive disorder have demonstrated that yoga helped them reduce their dosage of prescriptions or even got off them altogether. Not only will this save you money on medications but it reduces the likelihood of experiencing secondary effects and hazardous drug connections (be sure to consult your primary care physician before discontinuing or changing any recommended drugs).

Building mindfulness for change

Yoga and reflection help you cultivate mindfulness. Additionally, being more aware can make it easier to overcome negative emotions like outrage. Studies suggest that chronic annoyance and aggression are just as closely linked to coronary episodes as smoking, diabetes, and elevated cholesterol. Yoga appears to reduce outrage by deepening sensations of empathy and connection while quieting both the sensory system and brain. Yoga also enhances your capacity to step away from the drama of life, remaining resilient despite difficult news or life's ups and downs. While you don't need to respond immediately -- in fact, research has indicated that yoga actually speeds up response time! -- you can use that moment wisely and reduce longing over yourself or other people by choosing more thoughtful strategies.

Benefits Your Connections

Love may not solve all problems, but it sure can help with healing. Reassurance from family and friends has been shown time after time to promote wellbeing and recovery. Yoga practice itself cultivates benevolence, empathy, and greater poise - traits which might work on many of your connections as well.

Utilize sounds to relax your sinuses

Yoga offers many benefits, from asana and pranayama, to reflection. But there's more in its toolbox besides those. Consider reciting aloud; it will draw out exhalation which shifts focus toward the parasympathetic sensory system. When done in public, recitation can have a powerful physical and close-to-home impact. A new report from Sweden's

Karolinska Establishment suggests that murmuring sounds -- like those made while reciting Om -- open up sinuses and prevent seepage.

Guide your body's healing with your mind (mental benefits of yoga).

Visualizing a picture in your imagination, such as what is done during yoga Nidra or other practices, can bring about physical changes within yourself. Studies have found that directed symbolism lessened postoperative torment, reduced migraine recurrences, and enhanced personal satisfaction for individuals living with disease or HIV.

Kriyas, or cleansing practices, are another component of yoga. They encompass everything from rapid breathing exercises to deep internal cleansing of assimilation parcels. Jala neti, or sensitive lavage of nasal segments with salt water, wipes away residue and pollutants from the nose while keeping organic liquid away from creating and helping exhaust sinuses.

Helps You with Karma Yoga

Serving others is an integral part of yogic philosophy. Even if you don't feel inclined to serve others, doing so could potentially increase your prosperity in the long run. A survey at the School of Michigan found that those who contributed less than an hour a week were twice as likely to still be alive seven years later. Serving others gives meaning and perspective; your interests may not seem so pressing when you consider what others are making possible.

Upholds Self-Care

In much of traditional medicine, patients are treated as isolated recipients of care. Yoga helps you take control of your life by giving you tools for change - you could start feeling quite improved even after just one or two sessions with yoga! As with most things in life, the more committed you become, the greater benefits accrue. Engaging in yoga not only engages your thought processes; it gives you affiliation which empowers you to affect change; but trust itself can retouch.

Maintains Your Connective Tissue

As you read all of the ways yoga can benefit your wellbeing, it may have seemed like there was a lot of getting over. That's because they're intricately linked. Alter your position and it alters how you relax; alter your breathing pattern, it alters how tactile everything feels. This underlying principle underlies everything about yoga: Everything is connected - your hipbone to anklebone, nearby to world - this interconnection being essential for understanding yoga's effects. Plus, yoga utilizes various instruments which create additional substance and multiplicative effects! An enjoyable energy may just be the key ingredient responsible for healing all that yoga helps foster.

Chapter 16: What Is Yoga, And How Might It Benefit Me?

Yog is an ancient Indian practice that has evolved over centuries into a widely-used technique for monitoring physical and mental development. Although its origins remain obscure, its influence continues to spread today.

Yoga as practiced in the U.S. generally consists of authentic positions (asanas), breathing techniques (pranayama), and evaluation (Dyana).

Yoga offers a range of styles, from gentle to strenuous. When conducting research studies on its effects on achievement, researchers must take into account that each style may affect results. Therefore, it is important to clearly define and explore these influences when conducting studies on Yoga's benefits.

Yoga and two shows of Chinese start -- kendo and qi gong -- are commonly referred to as "shrewd new turn of events" practices. Each of the three practices incorporates both skillful parts and genuine ones.

Sherwin emphasizes the significance of "yoga," which derives from Sanskrit, as "association."

She believes this is an accurate depiction of Yoga in light of today's modern lifestyle: "We show it as unifying the mind and body through breathing exercises."

Sherwin emphasizes the many benefits of Yoga, noting its potential as a form of personal development. But Yoga is much more than that: "Yoga is an entire lifestyle," she states, noting its positions are only part of it. "Yoga is part of you!"

Yoga is an ancient Indian practice that has been practiced for thousands of years, according to Sherwin. "Initially," she states, "it was only shown one-on-one and only to men of great status," which today accounts for close to 5,000 years."

Yoga can be seen as a tool to cultivate success on all levels - physical, mental, basic and striking.

Yoga has yet to be subjected to many controversial convictions. According to The Yoga Connection, it will be regularly cleaned up and accepted by people of all beliefs, from realists and pundits alike.

History of Yoga

Yoga's approach to encounters often leaves gaps, including its oral transmission through texts and the perplexing thoughts of its models. Early works on Yoga were written on sensitive palm leaves which were eventually damaged, squashed or lost; some experts even speculate that Yoga may be as old as 10,000 years! Today we can trace Yoga's development back through four seasons of progress, practice and improvement - an illustrious past!

Pre-Standard Yoga

Yoga's roots were in Northern India's Indus-Sarasvati human progress. The word was first implied in the Vedas, sacred texts with tunes, mantras and customs for use by Brahmans - Vedic clergymen - who refined it further through Mystic diviners like Bhagavad-Gita (around 200 AD), one of the most notable Yogic game plans.

500 B.C.E. The Upanishads faced the challenge of custom appeasement from the Vedas and created a hybrid approach, emphasizing mental self-pictures through self-data, action (karma yoga) and data (jnana yoga).

Old Style Yoga

Prior to the advent of Patanjali's Yoga-Sutras, Yoga had been a patchwork of different beliefs and practices that often clashed. His text set the Standard timeframe for what we now refer to as "standard yoga," showing off its eight-limbed system which contained all aspects necessary for attaining Samadhi or illumination. Today, Patanjali is widely seen as the father of Yoga with his Yoga-Sutras still influential most styles today.

Post-Standard Yoga

Long after Patanjali, yoga masters developed practices designed to restore the body and bring out life. They disregarded the depictions of ancient Vedas and accepted that our body is an asset for reaching light. Tantra Yoga evolved out of these physical-amazing affiliations, using moderate thinking techniques to break through mental barriers that prevent us from being fully present in ourselves. This evaluation led us to develop Hatha Yoga as we know it today: body-focused practices with physical benefits.

The Present-Day Period

Yoga practitioners began making an impact in the late 1800s and mid-1900s, spreading their practices westward with students as both practitioners and followers. At the 1893 Parliament of Religions in Chicago, Expert Vivekananda mesmerized attendees with his discourses on Yoga and the diversity of world religions. In the 1920s and 30s, Hatha Yoga rose to a cult-like status in India thanks to T. Krishnamacharya, Expert Sivananda, and numerous yogis who practiced it. Krishnamacharya founded the pioneering Hatha Yoga school in Mysore in 1924, and Sivananda established his Incomparable Life Society on the banks of the holy Ganges Stream in 1936. Krishnamacharya left behind three students that would carry forward his legacy and spread Hatha Yoga: B.K.S Iyengar, T.K.V Desikachar, and PattabhiJois. Sivananda was an influential essayist, penning 200 books on Yoga while founding nine ashrams across nine different yoga bases around the world - from one side of India to the other.

Yoga's rapid spread towards the West began with Indra Devi opening her studio in Hollywood in 1947. Since then, more western and Indian educators have become pioneers of Hatha Yoga, inspiring countless fans and cultivating many schools or styles with various emphasises on preparation. Within a relatively short period, Hatha Yoga became ubiquitous across North America with numerous locations offering classes.

Importance and Benefits of Yoga

Over the years, there has been an upsurge in interest and understanding around Yoga. Clinical-trained experts and celebrities alike are endorsing its various advantages. While some see Yoga as simply another wide game plan with additional new age divination added on top, others find it quite bewildering that what they perceive to be just another action won't provide them with what they had originally hoped for.

Before we delve into the expected benefits of Yoga, it is essential to comprehend its true essence. Yoga isn't a religious practice but an approach for managing daily existence that cultivates a sound mind in a healthy body. Man is made up of physicality, mind, and infinite potential; Yoga serves as a bridge between these three aspects as taught in Ayurveda in India.

Certain kinds of action, such as uncharted territory, do not guarantee true prosperity. They generally lack any connection to the improvement or maintenance of one's physical or astral body.

Yoga is more than just bowing your body and holding the breath; it is an experience designed to bring you into a state where reality becomes your own reality and accepts everything as it is, giving life its true essence. Yoga allows for this connection between you and the universe as one cohesive unit - making all that one. This is the association created through Yoga: all things become one!

Guruji of Yoga, Patanjali, famously stated "Sthiramsukhamasanam," meaning a pose that brings out all your strength and flexibility. You may be shocked to know that an asana is only the start of what Yoga can offer; its goal is to bring harmony between all parts of yourself so you can achieve maximum benefit from all that exists within. Through

Yoga you will discover ways to bring out the best in yourself through self-acceptance.

Hatha Yoga and its various branches (Ashtanga Yoga, Iyengar Yoga, Bikram Yoga, Yin Yoga, Kundalini Yoga) can all provide harmony for those looking to achieve balance through preparation. Whatever suits you best depends on what you enjoy doing and the issues that need addressing during this practice.

Yoga offers many beneficial effects for health and fitness, such as:

* Expands frontal cortex limit

* Reduces tension impressions * Enhances quality explanation * Expands versatility

* Hacks downbeat

* Stretches lung capacity

* Combats fretfulness

* Moves unexpected back torture

* Further develops balance energy * Develop stronger bones * Strengthen weight bearing muscles

Cuts down the risk of heart illnesses:

Yoga as a status value has immense benefits that have an immense effect on people both physically and psychologically. From decreasing pulse rates to raising torment resistance, Yoga does many things well - just ask anyone!

Further Developed Course:

Yoga strengthens your bloodstream, leading to better oxygen transport throughout the body and improved skin radiance. Further strengthening this circulation system also promotes healthier organs and brighter complexions.

Further Establishes Position:

Yoga provides guidance on how to control and transform yourself physically. With regular practice, your body will eventually recognize the correct position, leaving you looking confident and balanced.

Hoists Your Personality:

Yoga helps hoist the personality into its proper place by teaching it how to relax into it. With regular practice comes automatic recognition of what needs changing! With standard practices you'll soon recognize where it needs changing!

Consistently practicing Yoga can awaken your spirit in a fleeting moment, filling you with invigorating energy.

Cut Down Circulatory Stress:

Regular yoga practice leads to improved blood circulation throughout your body. This promotes oxygenation of cells as there is a reduction in circulatory strain as your body relaxes.

Monitors Awkward Development:

Why not age gracefully and avoid early signs of aging? Yoga helps detoxify you, take out harm, and free radicals - not only that, but it also delays development too! Additionally, yoga recollects pressure which also has been known to slow down growth.

Reduces Strain:

While on your yoga mat, focus is placed on preparation. This ensures that all attention is directed toward the issue being discussed and your brain gradually releases any strain or bother that has been plaguing it.

A Drop in the Beat Rate:

Yoga works with your body by relieving strain. As your heart relaxes and opens up, your heartbeat rate decreases; this indicates your heart is functioning optimally and ready to pump more blood with fewer pounds on its back.

Increases Strength:

Your own body weight can help you build strength. This is an incredibly impressive method for strength building.

Anxiety The Board:

Bending, contorting and controlled breathing may assist with anxiety management.

Improve Cardiovascular Constancy:

Yoga increases oxygenation within the body and slows down the heartbeat, leading to higher cardiovascular constancy.

Lower Respiratory Rate:

Yoga involves controlled unwinding - filling your lungs with air so they can work more productively.

Fights Misery:

Yoga helps combat miserable feelings by channeling negative energy away. Even though you may feel hopeless, yoga helps channel that feeling of hopelessness into productive energy that helps combat misery.

Yoga Fosters Harmony:

Yoga not only seeks to create harmony in the classroom, but it also helps you manage your body. A typical demonstration of Yoga will focus on helping you adjust positions during class and concentrate outside the class as well.

Organ Care:

Yoga strengthens your internal organs, protecting you from contaminations. After some time has passed since practicing Yoga, however, if something doesn't feel quite right with your body after long preparation, then you must act quickly to determine why.

Yoga and Protection:

Yoga and opposition have long been connected. As Yoga strives to recover and develop each telephone in your body, your immunity increases significantly - strengthening it from within.

Yoga Invokes Full Body Care:

Doing yoga for personal reasons will help you develop awareness of your own body, enabling you to make small but significant changes that will improve how you live your life. With time, practicing yoga will lead to feeling good in yourself.

Enhancement in Gastrointestinal Prosperity:

Yoga regularly can benefit the stomach-related system and clear out other stomach illnesses like indigestion or gas. Plus, its abilities work for people of all ages; learn more about acid reflux home fixes here.

Extending Center Strength:

It is essential to recognize when your middle is solidified as well as when other parts of the body. Your center holds all the weight of your body, helping you recover more easily from wounds and increasing confidence in yourself. Yoga works on this area to make it sound, versatile and strong.

More Raised Degrees of Anguish Strength:

Yoga builds resistance against torture and helps alleviate ongoing distress.

Extended Absorption:

Yoga limits processing in order to achieve proper absorption - essential for reaching ideal weight.

Further developed Sexuality: Yoga encourages women to explore and embrace their sexuality without judgment or expectation of reward or punishment.

Yoga builds your courage and offers total release while increasing control. This gives your sexuality a vital lift.

Restored Energy:

Yoga can restore both mind and body to full functionality after regular practice. People who practice Yoga on a regular basis report feeling enabled after each gathering of Yoga poses.

Furthermore, practicing Yoga creates rest:

Yoga aids in completely relaxing your mind. It assists with working through unnecessary stresses, leading to better rest at night.

Composed Capacity of the Body:

Yoga encourages congruity. When you practice Yoga out of necessity, your mind begins to work in conjunction with your body, leading to improvement and magnificence.

Licenses Self-Affirmation:

Yoga encourages care and progress toward prosperity. Your confidence increases, making you more sure.

Promotes Self-Control:

Yoga shows you the best way to channel that caution into all areas of life.

Yoga Restores an Inspiring Perspective:

When practicing Yoga regularly, many aspects of your tactile system will be reset. This makes you more secure and allows you to look at life with a refreshed perspective.

Diminishing Enmity:

When yoga is practiced for any ordinary reason, its shock-absorption abilities are greatly improved. Deep breathing and examination calm the physical framework, decreasing irritation and hostility in its wake. A decline in hostility also implies a decrease in circulatory strain - leading to an overall more relaxed approach towards life.

Improve Concentration:

Consistent yoga practice will eventually bring about the best obsession and, after two to two months of consistent practice, you may find that you feel more prodded than ever before.

Quietness and Serenity:

Let your breath and thoughts engage you separately from each other, helping to reduce stress levels. Through regular yoga practice, you will discover how perfection becomes more than just an aspect of preparation - it becomes a way of life!

Nowadays, Yoga has become accessible to people of all ages and backgrounds. It has become part of everyday life for some and through electronic media has enabled yogis and educators around the world to share their expertise more than ever before.

Does Yoga Count as Exercise?

Although yoga wasn't originally created to be a movement program, some styles have evolved into practices focusing on its real components, according to Edward Laskowski MD - an experienced prescription and reclamation expert and former co-director of Mayo Office Sports Drug in Rochester, Minnesota. "People come into Yoga with different objectives. Some may do it just for fun or intellectual stimulation while others require more substantial action and development elements."

Dr. Laskowski emphasizes the importance of anything that increases our heartbeat during anticipation, as it can have a significant effect on overall wellbeing. "The heart is like a muscle," he states, noting that by exercising it with weights you make it stronger and more grounded." By grounding yourself physically with your pulse, Dr. Laskowski encourages us to keep moving towards positive experiences throughout our day.

Laskowski emphasizes that Yoga isn't quite on par with running or traveling when it comes to active pursuits. However, how much oxygen-consuming benefit one could derive from Yoga depends heavily on its style and pace, according to him.

Laskowski asserts that yoga can also aid in building mental fortitude. Certain positions and poses where an individual should hold up part of their body weight will challenge a muscle and help it become more grounded, according to Laskowski.

Yoga offers an effective strategy for getting your opponent situated, since its alignment of joints and muscle groups rather than supporting one particular muscle as in charge lifting would do, makes for more secure ground. "That is wonderful," according to Chan, "because that is exactly what we do in our everyday presence."

Clinical Benefits of Yoga

"Yoga has many benefits," Laskowski states. "Ultimately, it helps with adaptability, strength, interpersonal relations and endurance."

Research has demonstrated that stress reduction can help with various levels of success, such as weight loss support and cardiovascular wellness.

An analysis of one year's late evaluation data revealed that those who practiced Yoga experienced improvements across several dimensions of well-being, such as fear, stress, body structure, heartbeat rate and aggravation level in those with type 2 diabetes.

A meta-assessment revealed that yoga mediations could significantly reduce pulse rates among sensibly developed individuals with a B.M.I. of 25 or higher. The benefits were even more evident when the yoga intercession included breathing strategies and reflection.

According to another assessment, yoga motivated 66% of individuals to practice more and 40% to improve their eating habits.

There is evidence to support the idea that Yoga could benefit individuals suffering from chronic illnesses and infections, who endure torment or other adverse effects, as well as provide them with overall satisfaction.

Vinyasa Yoga

Vinyasa yoga is one of the most unique types of Yoga in America, according to Jen Fleming - yoga educator and supervisor at YogaWorks in Atlanta who was confirmed by Yoga Collusion. While vinyasa can often feel like an endless cycle of poses without progress like ashtangavinyasa does, her classes at Stream Vinyasa will be different as usual.

Vinyasa yoga styles such as power yoga, Baptiste yoga, Jivamukti and prana stream can be particularly intense and physically taxing, according to Fleming. Such classes tend to be among the most physically challenging for students.

Shala Worsley, a yoga educator at Who is Asheville Yoga Center in Asheville, North Carolina and certified by Yoga Plot, recommends that those new to vinyasa yoga try finding studios offering either an adolescent or tired stream class for some extra support. "Vinyasa can be quite fast-paced so if you don't have much experience yet with it then try finding an adolescent or exhausted stream class," she suggests.

Hot Yoga

Hot yoga cannot be replicated in a hotter room than what's offered at Healthwise Studios in New York City, according to Samantha Schupp - founder and educator at this hot yoga studio and certified by Yoga Plot. "Hot yoga cannot be performed the same way at each studio," she adds.

Schupp emphasizes the importance of taking into account all factors when planning a studio warming plan. Although temperature changes may be unique for each studio (check out your class diagram or call the specific studio to understand subtleties), the technique used can vary as well, she notes.

Nearby standard heating, two or three studios use humidifiers to make the space feel more humid. Healthwise also notes that some use infrared power from electric sheets put on top or around the room which may feel more regular than constrained air heat, Schupp states. Ultimately, Schupp notes, the size of the room, climate outside and how pressed a class is all factors in how bothersome a space becomes.

Hot Yoga Classes Aren't All Hot

"Warm Yoga," as the practice of Yoga in hot climates is commonly known, was popular in the 1970s with Bikram yoga style and power eventually played its part in modernizing various kinds of yoga styles.

Vinyasa or stream-type Yoga that is practiced in a heated studio may be referred to as hot Yoga. To maximize the benefit of such classes, Schupp recommends that students have some prior yoga experience before beginning them. Depending on the studio, an adolescent course might also be offered.

Pregnant Women, People With Heart Conditions, and Some Others Should Consult Their MD Before Doing Hot Yoga generally agree that yoga is safe for most healthy individuals in any time frame they are physically sound. However, Laskowski notes that those who have had significant medical issues in the past such as power injury or certain heart conditions, dry out easily or are pregnant may not be covered to do hot Yoga.

Laskowski advises that it's always wise to consult with a P.C.P. before undertaking any exercise that could put undue strain on your body.

What Are Other Popular Styles of Yoga?

According to Laskowski, there are approximately 20 basic varieties of Yoga. People often have various reasons and goals in mind when seeking to do Yoga, so he explains that there's no single answer for everyone when it comes to finding their bliss.

Based on your location and the size of the yoga community in your vicinity, you may find such yoga offered at studios near you. Here is a list of some local options.

Hatha Yoga

Hatha yoga (pronounced HAH-ta, not - that) encompasses various styles of Yoga such as ashtanga, vinyasa and power yoga. According to Fleming, Hatha classes tend to be slower-paced than their vinyasa counterparts and may not guarantee that each position will be followed immediately by another. Presents may be held for several breaths before moving onto another position, though one thing that remains constant across various kinds of Hatha Yoga is that positions should always relate to your breathing models.

Ashtanga Yoga

Ashtanga yoga is an intensely physical type of
Yoga that progresses rapidly from position to
position. Rather than streaming or vinyasa
Yoga, there are predetermined sets that must
be performed in a specific order. Ashtanga
can be taught either through instructor-led
classes or Mysore plans; Mysore allows the
teacher to present without actually leading
the class; understudies must memorize all
movements and timing from memory in these
latter cases, according to Fleming's
understanding.

Kundalini Yoga

Kundalini yoga combines positions, breathing,
reflection and the use of mantras. Ultimately,
kundalini yoga seeks to "blend" our inner
energies together while adding compassion.

Yin Yoga

Yin yoga is an active style where you remain
in one position for long periods of time before
moving onto another. You may choose to do

this on the floor, in your back or stomach, according to Fleming.

Fleming notes that uninvolved stretching is more uncomplicated and focused on expanding. Furthermore, positions are held longer than in other types of Yoga to promote joint health, according to Fleming. "This kind of stretching may actually be better for joints than dynamic growing," she adds.

Yoga Nidra

Yoga Nidra is more like an evaluation than a position-filled class. As the teacher guides them through loosening up various parts of the body, students lie on their backs (with or without support if desired). Yoga Nidra practitioners are encouraged to "let go" and surrender in order to relax and understand. According to Fleming, it could be just as resuscitating and accommodating as certified rest.

Basic Things Every Yoga Student Should Be Aware of

As you practice Yoga more frequently, the more positions you will learn. Everyone begins with a similar large pose; however, recent trends indicate that young adults are increasingly turning toward these adult poses which offer numerous benefits such as moving back torture, growing hips and creating congruency.

What You May Think About Yoga Mats -- and Other Yoga Props

A common misconception among some yogis is that props are only for novices or people who "are defective at yoga." But this couldn't be further from the truth; experienced yogis use props for various reasons, from comfort to making stretches safer if you have an issue or block, according to Tune Krucoff, a teacher accredited by both GRYA (General Relationship of Yoga Experts) and author of Yoga Shines: 108 Direct Practices for Strain Help in Seconds or Less.

Props can also be an essential element of class, like in seat yoga classes where most coordinated poses take place on a chair rather than the floor, according to Krucoff.

Yoga for Beginners: What You Ought to Know Before Your Five Star Retreat

Before embarking on any five star journey, here are some things you should be aware of:

Are you new to yoga? Before attending your first class, here is some important information that should be taken into consideration.

* Research the class thoroughly beforehand. Judi Bar, yoga expert and program boss at Cleveland Center Success and Preventive Medication, suggests that if a class appears juvenile, you might want to do further investigation. While children may be present, they may not have much desire to become five-star practitioners when taking lessons. "Junior classes tend to cater to extra young or fitter individuals or even those with little yoga experience," Bar advises. To be safe, speak with the teacher beforehand or watch some or all of the class before enrolling.

* If you're feeling particularly tired, Bar suggests trying a class for juveniles that encourages people to focus on their bodies. "On some erratic days," she advises, "it should feel kept up with in doing what feels comfortable," so don't worry about feeling like there's competition in the room if you're new at this.

* Engage with the teacher. Before class begins, get to know more about your teacher and share any memorable rates you've heard from other students. Laskowski recommends that if there are any wounds or innovative circumstances present in class, be sure to inform them as well; "Teachers are ready to assist with adjusting situations to reduce frustrating injury," he states. "Their support system will be invaluable during these trying times."

Take the necessary steps to not sweat the small stuff. Remember, everyone was once an adolescent at some point. "Yoga doesn't need to be complicated; no special dress or props is necessary; just an everyday clear practice," Sherwin advises. "Yoga should lead you towards discovering true concordance by then."

Fundamentals of Yoga

Yoga classes consist of many repetitive, physical activities called poses. Explanations on breathing patterns and reflection standards form the basis for any yoga class. When a position causes discomfort or appears hazardous, adjustments can be made with props like blocks, covers, lashes - even seats! Yoga isn't one-size-fits all: Your individual practice will depend on individual needs and goals.

Regular yoga practice offers numerous advantages. According to Roger Cole, Ph.D., a psychobiologist and certified Iyengar yoga educator, "yoga provides areas of strength that are fundamentally relaxing and reviving"; relaxation is built into every session."

Dr. Timothy McCall, author of "Yoga as Remedy," emphasizes the calming power of yoga's breath as a tool to help you become more in tune with your body and move more easily.

Recent studies have been increasingly emphasizing the medical benefits of Yoga.

* Decrease Back Torment: Yoga classes provide opportunities to relieve low back discomfort through optional impacts as well as regular extended get-togethers.

* Encourage Bone Thickness: In a recent study, yoga experts were found to have significantly thicker bones in their spine and hips compared to individuals in a benchmark bundle.

* Further developing balance: Male competitors in a lone report showed better congruency after 10 weeks of yoga classes than they did following an identical benchmark social event for competitors who didn't alter their schedules.

* Prevent mental debilitation: According to one study, those who combined yoga and reflection rather than just doing a brain arranging exercise performed much better on an assessment that measures visuospatial memory - essential for balance, critical thinking skillsets, and the capacity to perceive paradoxes and analyze the world more deeply.

* Reduced Stress: According to an assessment of 72 women, Iyengar yoga significantly reduced mental strain and the negative psychological and genuine consequences associated with strain.

* Reduce Misery: An assessment of coal excavators with reliable obstructive pneumonic sickness, or C.O.P.D., revealed that yoga could reduce weakness and tension levels.

Yoga Is Not New.

Yoga originated with an ancient Indian philosophy, so many poses in yoga classes have both Sanskrit and English names (for instance, adhomukhasvanasana is more commonly referred to as plunging facing canine pose). You might hear both names used interchangeably during class.

No matter if you have never taken a yoga class, you are already familiar with some of its concepts and practices. Have you ever done some poses in the air? That's what yoga is all about - getting fit!

Coaches and prosperity classes around the globe, along with school and most outstanding games social events, have begun incorporating Yoga into additional standard exercises as a means of strengthening mental focus, body molding, and helping competitors breathe better and focus better.

Yoga & Assessment

Yoga was long before it became a widely recognized physical activity; for much of its early history, it served primarily as an assessment practice.

Care with Yoga

In a yoga class, as you develop an efficient method for doing the poses, your instructor will likely instruct you to observe your breath and how your body moves during each activity. They cannot serve as the sole basis of creating a brain-body connection.

Yoga poses offer the unique opportunity to explore your entire body, encouraging you to pay attention to how each part feels as you progress through them. You might discover, for instance, that one side of your body feels different during a stretch than another, that changing up positions on one leg helps alleviate shoulder tension, or that certain pose helps ease push-ins in your neck.

Yoga transforms certain activities into tools to aid students in becoming more mindful and even developing an efficient method for reflecting.

Chapter 17: A Successful Strategy to Think About

Contemplating is an active process that offers rewards quickly. Here, we provide key advice to get you on your way toward more profound confirmation and contentment with life.

The Breath

Breathing strategies are an integral component of Yoga practice; not only do they help keep you on track while practicing, but they can also reduce strain, loosen the structure, and quiet the mind.

Elena Brower, a yoga and reflection educator and the creator of "Specialty of Thought," believes that Yoga breathing techniques provide an "open door to thought." According to Ms. Brower, more individuals who have recently discovered certified bits of Yoga are turning toward reflection as they recognize the value of having space to reflect, discharge and reset.

Next we explore breathing systems associated with yoga classes:

Stomach Loosening Up: Commonly known as diaphragmatic or waist breathing, this breathing technique is one of the most widely observed in yoga practice. It encourages clear, competent speaking that takes into account all factors.

Try it Out:

1. Inflate your middistrict as you inhale.

2. Exhale deeply to expel any air that might have entered your abdomen.

Ujjayi or "productive" breath: This form of deep inhaling allows you to slow and smooth out the flow of breath. It is often taught in stream classes to help students regulate their breathing while they move through positions.

Why not give it a try?

1. Squeeze the muscles at the back of your throat and inhale and exhale with your mouth closed.

2. Next, try this:

3. Inhale completely; 4 Release 33% of breath.

5 Pause. 6. Release another third of breath.

7 Pause and Exhale all remaining air from your lungs - 9 Repeat this cycle 5 more times for maximum effect

10. You may then opt to do some obstructed breathing during exhalation.

Substitute nostril relaxing: This strategy has been known to be successful at altering sensory system perception, so it's worth trying before contemplating.

Test it Out:

1. Seal one nostril shut and breathe in through the open one.

2. Exhale through this same nostril.

3. Switch hands and block off one nostril with your hand while keeping the other one open; inhale through this same open nostril and exhale out through it.

4. Do this several times until all are comfortable with how things feel in your nose. 5. Once comfortable with how things feel in your nose, repeat these steps several more times until your entire system feels relaxed and at ease.

Starting a yoga practice doesn't require anything special; however, you may find that certain items become helpful as your practice progresses.

No Socks, No Shoes - Absolutely No Issue

Yoga is often performed barefoot on a mat. Socks can be dangerous and should never be worn during yoga practice. If you must wear socks while practicing on your feet, look for sports socks with elastic grips on the soles for extra support and grip.

Yoga Mats

Most yoga studios and exercise centers provide mats; however, many yoga understudies prefer to purchase their own for cleanliness and the variety of materials, thickness, and tensile strength available. You might discover that certain kinds of mats provide greater support in certain areas than others.

Select a mat that will keep you from slipping and sliding, as this provides a secure platform for changing from pose to pose. Regularly clean your mat with antibacterial wipes; if renting mats at your studio or fitness center, bring along some small packages of antibacterial wipes for cleaning the rental mats.

Garments

Any exercise garments should suffice for yoga classes. However, clothing that is too baggy may cause problems as you progress into headstand and handstand poses.

Starting a Yoga Practice

Any attire suitable for yoga should be sufficient; any yoga garment can work perfectly well in the right circumstances.

To reap the full benefits of Yoga, it's essential to find a way to incorporate it into your regular practice.

Making a Habit

When starting any yoga practice (or any new wellness endeavor), remember that progress occurs by doing it regularly. Start small and achievable - 10 or 15 minutes of Yoga every day could be more beneficial than attending one class for seven days straight. As Dr. Phil once said, "I would prefer having an understudy succeed at doing one-minute-a-day practice than fail at doing five." Once you see the benefits of your daily regiment, chances are good that it will inspire more effort towards greater accomplishment over time.

Track Down a Class

Yoga can be done from home, but for beginners especially it's recommended to attend one or two classes taught by an experienced educator in either private or social settings. Doing this ensures your safety when practicing yoga practices.

When searching for a yoga educator, look for someone with at least 200-hour certification from an instructor certified with the Yoga Collusion. These projects should address injury preparation as well. If you have any clinical concerns, consult with a specialist before beginning to explore which types of Yoga might be most suitable for you.

If you are considering renting a yoga mat, search for yoga studios or rec centers that provide slip-safe mats and strong, clean blocks as backup. If you do decide to lease one, make sure there is access to an antibacterial shower or fabrics so you can wipe down your mat after use.

Do you need a tight center, strong arms, and defined legs? Grab your yoga mat and prepare to sweat! You'll be amazed at what you can accomplish.

What Class is Ideal for Me?

Yoga classes come in many different styles today. Some are challenging and will leave you sweating; others are delicate yet supportive. Some educators play music during class while others don't; some incorporate references to yoga reasoning or otherworldliness while others don't.

Here are a few types of classes your yoga studio or recreation center might provide:

Hatha: Today, most yoga styles that are being shown in America are of the Hatha variety. This term refers to the actual act of doing Yoga rather than reflection or reasoning about it. A Hatha yoga class typically consists of stances and breathing activities; however, its difficulty predicting whether they'll be challenging or delicate. Check with your school or educator for more information regarding classes exclusively labeled Hatha Yoga.

www.ingramcontent.com/pod-product-compliance
Lightning Source LLC
Chambersburg PA
CBHW062139020426
42335CB00013B/1263